# TAKING THE PLUNGE

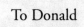

To Donald

# TAKING THE PLUNGE
## Swimming for Fitness

### BY PENNY CLARKE

**Illustrations by Raymond Turvey**

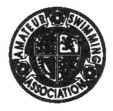

**Recommended by The Amateur Swimming Association**

BⓉXTREE

Before beginning this or any other fitness programme, always consult your doctor to make sure that it is suitable for your individual needs.

First published in Great Britain in 1994 by
Boxtree Limited · Broadwall House · 21 Broadwall · London SE1 9PL

10 9 8 7 6 5 4 3 2 1

ISBN: 185283 536 2

Text design by Martin Lovelock
Cover design by Robert Updegraff
Front cover photograph © David de Losey/The Image Bank
Back cover photograph: The Telegraph Colour Library

Printed and bound in Finland

A CIP catalogue entry for this book is available from the British Library

# CONTENTS

# ACKNOWLEDGEMENTS

My sincere thanks are due to many people for their help during writing this book: to my advisor Dr Dennis Rewt, Assistant Director of Physical Education at the University of Edinburgh, for his support, sense of humour and hilarious anecdotes; to John Lawton, Joan Harrison and Jackie Brayshaw of the Amateur Swimming Association, for their suggestions and comments on various drafts; to Debbie Figuerido, ASA Synchro Coach and Sports Development Officer for Westminster City Council, for her ideas and enthusiasm on Chapter 10; to Lisa Davies and Andy Sprod, for their story of swimming monks; to Arthur Stewart, Lecturer at the PE Department of the University of Edinburgh, for his advice on open-water swimming and safety; to Anne Kennett of the Royal School of Veterinary Studies, and the staff of the Erskine Medical Library and Main Library at the University of Edinburgh, for helping us dig up information; to Raymond Turvey for his brilliant illustrations, and to Wanda Whiteley and all the staff at Boxtree, for making this book such a painless experience; and last, but by no means least, to my long-suffering sister Sarah. As researcher for this book, her tireless pursuit of the weird and wonderful went above and beyond the call of duty, while her ideas and patience can only be marvelled at. Thanks.

# INTRODUCING WATER

*Taking the Plunge* is about an elemental medium which has enchanted people since the earliest times. It's about an environment whose properties remove the crunch from high-impact workouts; which supports movement where disability inhibits; which enhances relaxation and helps rehabilitation. It's about exhilarating challenge and soothing rest; new-fangled technology and age-old therapies. It's about having a go, and keeping on going: about getting in there, getting wet and getting on with it.

Water – the very essence of life. We drink it. We bathe in it. We trust it as a symbol of purity and we're lured to it as a symbol of sex and rejuvenation. It's familiar yet it's exciting, an image of natural innocence and elemental passion. It is, quite simply, the most inspiring substance around, supporting life as well as enhancing it

*Taking the Plunge* takes a fresh look at all water has to offer as an approach to fitness which is so varied, so dynamic and so effective you'll wonder why you ever stagnated on dry land.

● It provides practical advice and step-by-step instructions on using water as a natural gymnasium.

*But it's not just an aquafit workout.*

● It helps you feel more at home in the pool and improves your stroke technique.

*But it's not just a swimming manual.*

● And from freezing baths to soothing spas, it takes a refreshing look at all the different water treatments available.

*But it's not just a book about hydrotherapy.*

*Taking the Plunge* is about making the most of water. From the shores of Korea to the seductive solitude of flotation tanks, it'll whet your appetite and inspire you to go along to your local pool to become part of an approach to health and fitness which reaches back through the ages to the very beginnings of time. Because *Taking the Plunge* even leaves you wondering about our evolution into human beings – about why our bodies are designed the way they are; why we feel such a magical attraction to such a simple substance; and whether we really are far more adapted to the sensual environment of water than we could ever have imagined …

Exercise should be no big deal – just a few short minutes amidst the rush of everyday life when you can do something you actively enjoy.

Can it make the difference for you? Take the plunge and find out.

# Part One

# TESTING THE WATER

# Chapter 1

# EQUIPMENT
## From Suits to Kick Sticks

'It is impossible to find costumes which are modestly cut, still in attractive colours, and not made for the larger person. Petite, slim women don't necessarily want to parade around the pool as though in a beauty pageant ...'

Letter, *Sport and Leisure*, November/December 1992

When all you actually need to take the plunge is some water and a swimsuit of some description, it is ironic that this book begins by looking at all the different water equipment now on offer. After all, in this 'natural gymnasium', so perfectly adaptable to so many different needs, what could be more liberating, what more invigorating than the wonderful simplicity of water and skin? But then again, more and more is being made of water, intensifying the results while losing nothing of the natural, uncluttered enjoyment it provides. And a quick dive through the history of modern swimwear, for instance, will show you why the design of your cozzy could well add considerably to this enjoyment.

> The Australian Dawn Fraser claimed she could have broken every record in the book if allowed to swim naked. Nudity originated in the Greek Olympics when Orsippus dropped his loin-cloth and was seen to gain a distinct advantage ...
>
> Charles Sprawson, *Haunts of the Black Masseur*

in the 1920s, right up until the late 1950s, light, quick-drying silk was the favoured material. But then Speedo introduced their new water-repellent costumes made from nylon, and this material remained popular until the early 1970s when Lycra set out to become the household word it is today.

# Togs – Great and Small

Swimming gear – male and female – has evolved steadily over the years. During the development of international competition

### Go-faster fabrics
However, the pace of development hasn't stopped there. The 1992 Olympics saw the launch of the latest revolutionary competition cozzy – Speedo's suitably techno-sounding S2000, 'scientifically developed ... [with] unique flatlock

stitching with a significant 15 per cent reduction in water drag co-efficient ... an ergonomic 'second skin' for maximum hydro-dynamic performance and ease of stroke movement ... [producing] record breaking results ...'

And just a year later, Arena's Swim Tech '96 became the splash hit at the European Swimming Championships in Sheffield. Weighing no more than a pair of nylon tights, both these new costumes are so thin that they have to be black for the sake of modesty, and their design steps away from a scooped neckline in favour of a high turtle that has to be pulled on over the head and fastened teddy-like at the gusset. The result? A fit so tight that not even air bubbles can get trapped between your body and the highly elastic Lycra-polyamid combination, a material reported to have a lower water resistance than skin. So while in the past top-class swimmers had no option but to shave off their body hair if they wanted to improve their race times, today's costumes cut water resistance to a minimum. Resistance from men, however, is proving harder to overcome. The prospect of wearing a full swimsuit is less appealing than conventional skimpy trunks, it seems.

## Feel the fit

Of course, the desire to shave a hundredth of a second off a world record is not something that really affects the likes of you and me – especially at the present cost of at least £60 a suit. But it might be an idea to think about the design principles involved, as they do affect us when choosing our swimwear.

Baggy boxers are out. Not only will the spectacle of bobbing manhood leave people gasping in your wake, but the more fabric your trunks use, the greater the water resistance you encounter – making light, closely fitting swimwear which restricts movement as little as possible the only choice for both men and women. Needless to say, bikinis are also a bad idea, unless you plan on exercising with one hand holding up your drawers, and if you're taking part in an aquafit class, a support top or sports bra underneath your costume is highly recommended. After all, you'd never dream of going to an aerobics class and letting it all bounce free, and as your top half won't always be in the water, the effect can be just as uncomfortable in an aquafit workout.

---

If you do find your costume rubs for any reason, a touch of Vaseline does wonders.

---

Indeed, as technology marches on apace, and the fitness industry continues to blossom, specific aquafit gear reflecting the leotards and cycling shorts of land-based aerobics classes is rapidly gaining popularity. And if that isn't enough, Speedo are working on yet another type of fabric – one which does the opposite of the modern swimwear described above and holds water to make you work even harder by increasing your drag (see page 24).

And the future? According to Sue Tomkinson's article in *Aerobics and Fitness World* of June 1993, even the age-old excuse that it's too cold to strip off will soon no longer wash. Speedo have yet another secret formula up their sleeve – a swimsuit which actually retains body heat and keeps you warm. Of course, if they could design a costume which did the workout for you, that really would be impressive.

With your swimsuit sorted out, however, and a refreshing plunge just moments away, there's one last piece of equipment you should think about.

# 'The Compleat Goggler'

The 1930s' manual on underwater swimming which used this as a chapter heading must have conjured up a bizarre vision indeed for its contemporary readership. Today, however, goggles are probably the only other essential item for your swimming shopping list – to protect your eyes and help you see more clearly in the pool.

## Blurred at the edges

Even if the water is clear and the lighting is excellent, your vision will still be limited once you dip your face under the surface because light waves bend differently in water than they do in air – reducing your focus by a factor of 10. If you place a pocket of air between cornea and water, however, your eyes can focus again – exactly what happens when you put on goggles.

## Water contacts

And things are even looking brighter for people wearing contact lenses, as a recent paper in *Optometry and Vision Science* points out. Josephson and Caffery's survey of the factors involved in wearing contacts in water (1991) shows that swimming and hydrogel or soft lenses *can* mix. And not only can these be worn

behind masks and goggles, there are several ways of minimizing the risk of ocular infection as well. The paper also provides a few useful tips on preventing lenses from floating off when working out – like putting them in about half an hour before entering the pool, or inserting a couple of drops of *sterile* distilled water into the eye. It goes without saying, however, that you should seek your optician's advice before jumping in.

## The sting

For many people, though, it's not clarity of vision that's important for an enjoyable swim, but avoiding the sting. Water has a different pH (acidity–alkalinity) from the body's natural fluids, making it uncomfortable for some people to open their eyes when submerged. And while the use of other less stringent disinfectants like sodium hypochloride and iodine is now becoming more widespread, for many years chlorine was the only option. Although chloride is one of our body's natural salts, it can irritate the eyes when combined with the nitrogen and ammonia in the water, and regular swimmers may even see halos and rainbows around pool lighting if they develop a chlorine sensitivity.

▲ Alcohol makes your eyes even more sensitive to chlorine – one of many reasons why you should never mix drinking with water.

Of course, chlorine tolerance varies from individual to individual, and, according to Josephson and Caffery's survey, wearers of hydrogel contact lenses have the advantage here, as the lenses actually protect the eyes. Either way, though, if your local pool still uses this method of disinfectant, any irritation you may feel is only ever short-lived and can be eased by bathing the eyes gently in tap water.

## Don't get all steamed up

As with costumes, there is a huge range of goggles available on the market today, and your choice will ultimately be dictated by the fit and the price you wish to pay. Once adjusted properly, however, the next problem is to prevent them from steaming up. There's nothing sinister about this happening as the condensation is simply due to your skin temperature being warmer than the water in which you're working. Some goggles now come with the promise of patented anti-fog coatings – although in my experience this only lasts for the first few trips to the pool – but whichever type you choose, there are many other tricks of the trade to keep your vision clear.

Spitting into the goggles and wiping the saliva around the inside of the eyepieces is a popular choice, as is putting the goggles on dry rather than dunking them into the pool before you set off. Alternatively, you can always smear a little liquid detergent around the insides when you're in the changing-room, producing a film over the plastic to prevent beads of condensation forming. It's a lot less expensive than the commercial products used in diving masks, motorcycle helmets and on rifle sights.

▲ Take care when putting goggles on and taking them off. Always place the eyepieces over the eyes first before stretching the elastic around the back of your head. Otherwise it's all too easy for the goggles to ping back into your face.

# Optional Extras

### To cap it all

While healthy, intact skin will not be affected by lengthy exposure to chlorine, everyone knows that it doesn't do your hair a whole lot of good. One way of counteracting this is to use the ASA-endorsed Ultraswim products designed to release the chlorine bonds which attach to the strands. Alternatively, there are always swimming caps – providing, that is, you can find one that fits properly – and should you ever reach competition standard, they are a much less drastic way of streamlining your body than shaving your head, not to mention providing triathletes who swim in open water with a valuable source of insulation.

> Some 30 per cent of your body heat is lost through your head, so it makes sense to insulate this small area properly rather than adding extra layers elsewhere.

### Ear, nose and throat

For people who find it difficult to balance the pressure of air and water in the ears, individually moulded ear plugs are available. Always make sure your ears are dry and warm before inserting them, though, and should you get any sort of ear infection, avoid their use – and stay out of the pool until it's cleared up.

▲ Never wear ear plugs when diving.

Nose clips, on the other hand, are used

to balance the pressure in the nasal passages and protect the sensitive membranes at the back of the throat. They may look ridiculous, but they're essential for all synchronized swimmers and some competitive divers too (see Chapter 9).

## Aquatic intensity

And if you want to improve your swimming technique and increase the demand of your workout? Look no further than the traditional floats and hand paddles available on request at your local pool. Take kickboards, for instance. Indispensable if you wish to improve your leg and arm action in all strokes, they can also be incorporated into your aquafit routine as well – for instance, sweeping them sideways under the surface to increase your upper body strength. And pool buoys? These are floats you grip between your thighs to improve your body position when swimming, but they can also be used to tone up the chest and the backs of the arms by pressing them slowly downwards beneath the water surface.

And if you're allowed to use it – *and know how to use it properly* – the range of

> Take two bladders, blow them full of wind, and fasten them so together, that [you] may have them to lie under [your] armholes: which will easily bear [you] up.
> *The Art of Swimming*,
> Master Everard Digby, 1587

new aquafit equipment designed to increase resistance, buoyancy and weight in your workout is vast. For instance, Hydro-Tone's natty Hydro-Boots are a

must in aquatic footwear – water's answer to ski-boots for the ultimate in low-impact workouts. And if you're recovering from injury or simply want an extremely demanding workout, foam-filled exercise belts like the Aquajogger by Vulkan UK provide the slightly strange option of deep-water running – where your feet never even touch the bottom!

---

Leonardo da Vinci reputedly designed the first-ever flippers.

---

Needless to say, the selection is just as wide for swimmers being coached to competition standard. Harrington Products' Kick Stick, for instance, is a brace-like training device which ensures that you not only kick from the hip in front and back crawl, but point your toes on the downward action to promote ankle flexibility and a feel for the water. And if underwater microphones and receivers are a little excessive, and waterproof heart-rate monitors not your thing, you can be coached on the latest in swim benches instead, allowing you to practise your pulls and correct body alignment without even having to get wet.

Water needs no additives, and there's already enough variety in the different forms of aquatic exercise without getting hung up on technology. You don't need go-faster fabric to slice effortlessly up the pool, and you can make enough of a splash in an aquafit class without any new gadgets. But if you do get hooked and wish to supplement your efforts, it's all there for the taking. But then again: you won't know what you're missing if you don't take the plunge.

Benjamin Franklin, pioneer of American independence, designed the first hand-paddles which are now a standard feature of all swimming classes: 'I remember I swam faster with the use of these palletes but they fatigued my wrists.'

▲ None of the aquafit exercises in Chapter 6 use any devices to increase intensity. But if you do decide to take things a stage further, always make sure that you are confident with the given movement first, that you are properly supervised when trying it out, and that you increase the intensity gradually, making doubly sure that your technique and body alignment are perfect at all times and that you 'place' the equipment carefully rather than flinging it about wildly. And never use any added extras without warming up thoroughly beforehand, or cooling down and stretching out properly afterwards.

# Chapter 2

# THUMBS UP FOR WATER FITNESS
## Essentials for Enjoyment

Water fitness leads the way in terms of injury-free participation, according to a survey carried out by D. Weightman and R. C. Brown for the *British Journal of Sports Medicine* in 1979 – a fact not to be taken lightly. Apart from being a real pain, injury means you can't continue to exercise; and if you can't exercise, you can't continue improving your level of fitness. So there's more than one reason why safety makes sense.

## Playing the Game

All games have rules, and the fitness game is no exception. We all want to work out safely and in a way which gets results, and most people already know that there are guidelines set down to make exercise programmes as rewarding as possible. So here's a quick refresher course ... in case you've forgotten.

## Check it Out

Before embarking on any form of fitness programme, *everyone* should pop along to their doctor and make sure that it's appropriate for them. Water is a unique medium in that people with all kinds of

Injure yourself in football, rugby or squash, and nobody bats an eyelid. Injure yourself following some form of personal fitness programme, and you're likely to end up at the centre of the latest media scare story.

disabilities and medical problems can exercise effectively under supervision, but common sense will tell you that if you have, say, a cardiac or respiratory complaint, suffer from frequent dizzy spells, high blood pressure or a bone or joint problem like arthritis which might be aggravated by exercise, if you are pregnant or are on any kind of medication other than the contraceptive pill – *check it out first* ... even if you're over 50 and feeling great, but simply haven't had a workout for a while.

And once you've got the thumbs up, remember:

● Feel good. Although you probably won't want to exercise if you are unwell, do not enter the pool if you have had flu or any kind of cold or fever within the last 48 hours – or, indeed, have a skin infection, open wound or diarrhoea. You won't be the only person who'll feel worse for your efforts. Other people will too.

● Never hurt. There's a big difference between the sensation of a muscle or body part being worked, and that muscle or body part feeling painful, so stop the movement immediately if it doesn't feel right and go back to pulsing gently on the spot (see page 30). If the pain continues, seek medical advice.

● Drink before, during and after your workout – despite your fluid environment. Thirst is an inaccurate indicator of how dehydrated you may be. Don't drink alcohol, of course.

▲ Let buoyancy raise your spirits. Pre-swim alcohol can be lethal.

● Food and exercise – they don't mix! Wait

Cramp is simply an involuntary but acute muscular contraction. And while popular mythology advocates the consumption of salt or so-called electrolytic drinks, this connection has yet to be proved – and anyway, they might not be available when needed. Instead, simply relax, leave the water if you can, and do a gentle, static stretch on the muscle in question lasting up to a full minute (see chapter 7).

at least an hour and a half after eating anything before entering the water. You have to give your body a chance to begin the digestive process, because it might not be cramp that affects you but nausea – even vomiting.

Although we often think of 'fitness' as one item, it's actually a combination of many different attributes. And these can be roughly divided into those which improve our overall health – cardiovascular (aerobic) fitness, muscular strength and endurance, flexibility and body composition – and those which relate to our ability to perform different activities – skills like co-ordination, balance, power, speed and so forth, all of which you'll develop as you perfect your swimming and aquafit technique.

# Making the Most of Exercise

Of course, it would be great if the very act of immersion got us 'fit'. But miraculous though it is, even water can't do that for you, and while Chapter 14 shows that immersion can have a profoundly therapeutic effect on our bodies, there are a few simple things we have to bear in mind if we want to get results.

● Try to do some form of exercise at least three times a week, not necessarily just in the water, but anything which gets your heart pumping – even just a brisk walk to work in the morning.

Balance productive exercise with well-earned rest. Fitness is the *key* to a healthy life – not an alternative or substitute.

Indeed, 'cross training' – the mix-and-match approach to exercise – not only prevents that most dangerous of conditions, boredom, but has the advantage of making a whole range of different demands on your body so that it improves in a range of different ways.

● Aim to exercise for at least 20 minutes without stopping – although if it's been a while since you were last in circulation, make this your goal, and work up to it gradually.

Don't set yourself up to fail. Aim for too much too quickly and you'll only be disappointed.

● Remember to warm up, cool down and stretch out properly each time you exercise

Exercise regularly, and not only will your body burn up more energy than normal during the workouts themselves, but your whole metabolic rate will start to increase so that you burn up more energy more of the time – even when you're watching TV!

(see Part Two).

● Check your heart! The more times a minute it beats, the harder you are working. So monitor your heart rate (HR) regularly by placing two fingers just below the back of your jaw bone *on one side*, or just on the outside edge of your upturned wrist.

The following table shows you the number of beats per minute (bpm) you should be aiming at, as well as giving you this number calculated over a 10-second count for simplicity's sake. It's called your 'training zone', and is between 60 and 85

## Heart Rates for Landbased and Aquatic Exercise

| AGE | TRAINING ZONES | | | |
|---|---|---|---|---|
| | Beats per minute (60–85 per cent) | | Beats per 10 seconds (60–85 per cent) | |
| | Land-based exercise | Aquatic exercise | Land-based exercise | Aquatic exercise |
| 20 | 120 – 170 | 103 – 153 | 20 – 28 | 17 – 26 |
| 25 | 117 – 166 | 100 – 149 | 20 – 28 | 17 – 25 |
| 30 | 114 – 162 | 97 – 145 | 19 – 27 | 16 – 24 |
| 35 | 111 – 157 | 94 – 140 | 19 – 26 | 16 – 23 |
| 40 | 108 – 153 | 91 – 136 | 18 – 26 | 15 – 23 |
| 45 | 105 – 149 | 88 – 132 | 18 – 25 | 15 – 22 |
| 50 | 102 – 145 | 85 – 128 | 17 – 24 | 14 – 21 |
| 55 | 99 – 140 | 82 – 123 | 17 – 23 | 14 – 21 |
| 60 | 96 – 136 | 79 – 119 | 16 – 23 | 13 – 20 |

per cent of the maximum number of bpm your heart can *theoretically* achieve.

▲ BE SENSIBLE. If you have not exercised for a while, are over 50 years of age, or have some sort of medical condition likely to be aggravated by this level of intensity, aim to work at the lower end of the zones shown in this chart. And if you are on any sort of medication, check with your doctor first because this could also affect your HR.

● 'Aquatic HRs'. One of the bonuses of working out in water is that your whole circulation actually works more efficiently, your heart having to beat fewer times per minute to pump the blood around your body. So do be aware that other factors are at large once you begin exercising in the pool, and that the traditional HRs for land-based workouts should be seen as the *absolute maximums*.

---

Keep talking! If you work 'somewhat hard' to 'hard', and can still carry on a conversation – you've got it right!

---

● Gradually try to push yourself just that little bit more than you did the last time so that your body adapts to the new demands.
● And remember: if you don't use your

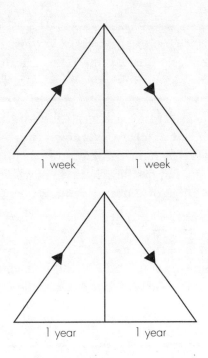

fitness, you lose it, the simple pyramids above showing you just how quickly this can happen.

Yet another good reason to opt for a sustainable approach to exercise – one which fits into your lifestyle naturally, which you look forward to and enjoy rather than thinking of as a chore.

---

For some additional guidelines for exercise during pregnancy, see Chapter 8.

# Chapter 3

# FLOATS, LIFT AND ALL THAT DRAG
## A Little Drop of Aquaphysics

Part of water's magical allure is the change you feel the moment you immerse yourself. You enter a world where gravity seems to disappear, where your movements are slowed and bearing more graceful, where buoyancy keeps you up while resistance holds you back, and where knowing *why* things react so differently helps you make your actions that much more effective. So whether exercising on it, in it, under or through it, *Taking the Plunge* gets your feet wet with a little drop of aquaphysics.

## Upwardly Mobile

No matter how well adapted to water we are, no matter how strong at swimming or how expert at life-saving, which of us hasn't stepped back at some point in our life and imagined the unimaginable: slowly sinking down to the bottom and never coming up. But then again, if iron and steel can remain at the surface when hammered thin and beaten into shape, it's a fair bet that even the down-and-out 'sinkers' in our midsts will be able to

---

Sinker – one adult male in 20 who finds buoyancy a let-down.

---

The human body is about 70 per cent water, an amount temporarily increased through drinking and also immersion – the 'pruny' effect on fingers and toes when you bathe being the result of your skin absorbing a small amount more.

float – with a little extra lift where it matters most.

### Women on top
On the whole, women tend to have less of the dense muscle tissue covering their frames than men and more of the dreaded body fat. But far from being a cruel fact of life, it actually means women have a clear advantage when working out with water.

Not only do women tend to float higher

> Average body-fat percentages reported for swimmers are about 7 per cent for males and 19 per cent for females … well below the normal values of 15 per cent and 25 per cent for males and females respectively.
>
> Thomas Reilly, 'Swimming', *Physiology of Sports*

than men, but this comforting layer around the hips, stomach and thighs also allows a more streamlined position in the water by helping to keep the lower half from sinking. The result? It costs women about 30 per cent less energy than men to swim a given distance. Or to put it another way, women can swim faster than men using the same amount of energy (McCardle, Katch and Katch, *Exercise Physiology*, 1991), one of the reasons why the difference in performance between the sexes is less in swimming than in other sports – by 1980 a mere 5 per cent separating the men and women's 400m freestyle world records (Allen Guttmann, *Women's Sports*) – and a factor which comes increasingly into play as the distances get longer.

---

The current record for swimming the English Channel is held by a woman.

---

So is there no hope for sinkers? Far from it, because body fat isn't the only thing keeping us afloat. By far the most important factor of all in controlling our buoyancy is the air in our lungs.

The floats and basic skills which follow are the type of things you'll practise when you go on any swimming course. Remember, *Taking the Plunge* is not designed to teach anyone to swim from scratch, but to refresh the memory and provide useful tips on stroke improvement (see Part Three). And if it does inspire you to go on a swimming course at your local pool, so much the better. Learning in a group is great fun, and you'll have a laugh getting feedback from your instructor, perfecting your skills and techniques all the more quickly .

▲ Make sure you read the advice in Chapter 3 before entering the water.

## Back float

Standing in chest-deep water, fill your lungs with a good deep breath so that your rib-cage lifts. Let your arms float out naturally at each side and gently lean backwards, eyes up to the ceiling, so that the back of your head enters the water as your feet leave the floor. Let your head find its own level – probably with the water just covering your ears – and relax, with your arms floating above shoulder-height.

You'll probably find that your feet stay low in the water, so think about lifting your hips and keeping those lungs filled with air. You are actually balancing in the water around your lungs – the body's natural centre of buoyancy (COB), which

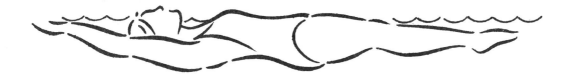

is located a couple of inches higher than your centre of gravity (COG).

---

*The more relaxed you are, the better you'll float.*

---

Now gently raise your arms above your head. Your COB immediately changes to balance your legs better so that they lift in the water to improve your float.

And now draw your arms down to your sides and feel the difference as your feet sink and you float almost vertically.

If you're not too confident in the water yet, an alternative is to try this at the edge of the pool by holding on to the side with one hand. Bend your knees, lower your shoulders into the water and, taking a deep breath, gently look directly upwards so that the back of your head is in the water. You will be floating parallel to the wall.

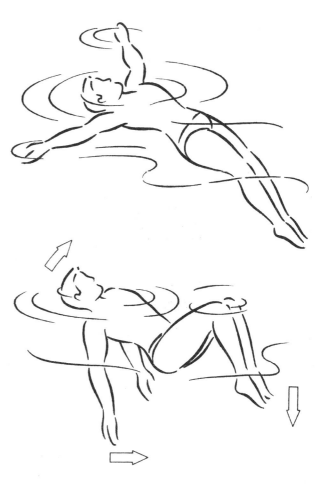

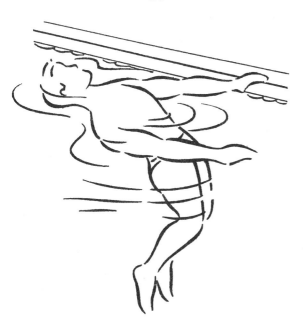

### Standing up – from your back

To regain your footing, scoop both hands firmly downwards and forwards towards your toes. Simply tuck your chin in so that your head lifts, draw your knees in towards your chest until you're in a sitting position, and then lower your feet to the bottom of the pool.

● Keep your shoulders in the water at all times.

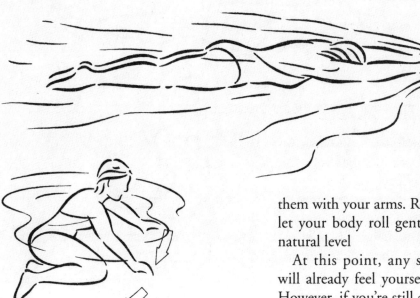

## Standing up – from your front

And it's the same idea if you're on your front. Tuck your knees in again and press your hands downwards and backwards towards your toes as you once more lift your head and lower your feet to the bottom.

## Mushroom float

Back to floating again, the mushroom float's a bit of a face-wetter, testing your body's natural buoyancy while getting you used to breathing out through your nose and mouth underwater as well. Standing once again in waist-deep water, this time take a deep breath, tuck your chin under so that your face is submerged, and tuck your knees into your chest, supporting

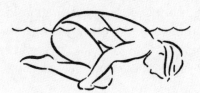

them with your arms. Relax once more, and let your body roll gently until it finds its natural level

At this point, any sinkers among you will already feel yourselves begin to drop. However, if you're still afloat, exhale slowly through both mouth and nose and feel yourself gradually sink beneath the surface. Uncurl whenever you're ready, drop your feet to the floor and stand up again.

Simple techniques to get your feet wet. But it's not just in swimming that buoyancy comes into its own – it's also one of the reasons why aquatic exercise is such a safe and effective approach to fitness.

# Safe but Sound

In shoulder-deep water you experience 90 per cent apparent weight loss.

Gravity may well keep your feet on the ground, but it also squeezes your joints together like a concertina. Once you are immersed in chest-deep water, however, your major joints lift and separate slightly, allowing better circulation and a greater range of movement. Those jolting, jarring impact forces compressing your ankles, knees, hips and lower back in land-based

> The squeeze and massaging effect we experience in water may be one of the reasons why we seem to need to pee more often when we exercise in the pool than on terra firma.

exercise all but disappear. The risk of injury plunges dramatically, and you can exercise safely for far longer.

But there's more, because the combination of buoyancy and water pressure can have a profound effect on your circulation too. Supporting and gently massaging the body, this hydrostatic squeeze is thought to aid the blood-flow from the lower limbs, actually playing a part in keeping your heart rate down (see page 18). You get the same CV benefits as on dry land but with far less stress on that most crucial of muscles.

And while we're talking muscles, water fitness is unique for another very important reason: muscle balance.

## Muscle action

> There are an amazing 792 muscles in the human body.

Every time you move, every time you perform even the simplest of activities, your body engages in a complex sequence

> 'Strength' is the ability of a muscle or muscle group to overcome a resistance or exert a force. 'Endurance' is its ability to carry out less intense activity over a longer period of time.

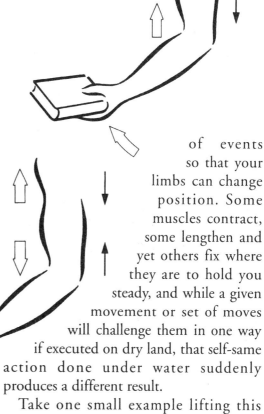

of events so that your limbs can change position. Some muscles contract, some lengthen and yet others fix where they are to hold you steady, and while a given movement or set of moves will challenge them in one way if executed on dry land, that self-same action done under water suddenly produces a different result.

Take one small example lifting this book: as you slowly raise the book up, the biceps muscle in front of your arm steadily shortens against both the book's weight and the pull of gravity ('con-centric' contraction), leaving the *opposing* muscle group *behind* your arm – your triceps – no option but to lengthen. Place the book on the table again, and to stop your hand falling straight down, that same biceps muscle gradually lengthens once more to control the movement against the pull of gravity ('eccentric' contraction) – your triceps again having no choice but to return to its shortened state. In other words, your biceps does all the work.

## The aquafit challenge

If you try this exercise in water, however, taking most of the gravity away and replacing it with buoyancy and the other forces operating under the surface, the balance between the work carried out by your biceps and triceps in this action changes. Not only will your biceps have to work harder to raise your hand against the surrounding water, but in order to lower it again you actually have to press down quite hard. And this pressing action means that your triceps must *actively* contract against the resistance to bring about the movement. *Both* muscles are worked evenly by one simple exercise, making their action balanced and saving you the trouble of having to do two separate exercises to strengthen your upper arm. Perfect.

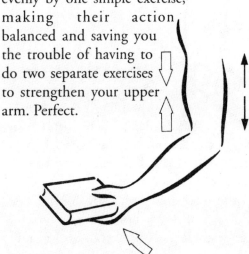

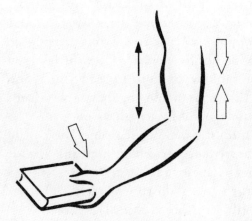

# Resistance, and All That Drag

> [Olympic champion Murray] Rose described the immediate sensual awareness of water as he dived in, the feeling that he was suspended, united with the element, the sudden surge of power like that experienced by ballet dancers who remove their hair to activate their nerve-endings ... Shaving has become a complex science. The secret is not to overdo the shaving or the thrill is lost, to restrain the shaves so more hair comes off when required.
>
> Charles Sprawson, *Haunts of the Black Masseur*

Whether or not the removal of body hair does something for your nerve endings, the issue at stake here is water resistance – swimmers at Murray Rose's level of performance trying to reduce any unnecessary drag which body hair might create. But resistance is also what allows you to move through the water in the first place, as well as placing a demand on your body during your aquafit workout.

## Aquatic exercise and drag

> Increase the amount of surface area you present to the water and you increase the resistance you encounter. Compare, for instance, how exhausting it feels when walking or jogging through chest-deep water, with the energy-efficient streamlining achieved by good swimming technique.

Aquafit is all about *maximizing* the effects of any forces which *inhibit* your progress through the water so that you increase the intensity of your workout. Part Two provides an aquacircuit which you can adapt to your individual level of fitness.

## Swimming and drag

Swimming, on the other hand, is all about *minimizing* the effects of any forces which resist your progress through the water, and capitalizing on those which propel you forwards. In other words, you should try to be as streamlined as possible when you swim, holding a steady horizontal position while using your arms, and particularly your hands, to 'catch' the water and pull your body forwards.

### 'Catching' water

1. Palm facing your body, and fingers pointing vertically downwards in the water, slice your hand backwards through the water leading with your little finger.
2. Now rotate your wrist so that your palm faces backwards and repeat the movement.
3. Open your fingers and try this again.

4. And once more with your fingers together and your hand slightly cupped.

The difference in resistance you feel each time should be quite marked, and when swimming, you want to be able to grab hold of as much water as possible so that your pull is as strong and effective as you can make it.

After all, 'every action has an equal and opposite reaction.' Or to put it another way:
● if you pull backwards and downwards in the front crawl, you propel yourself forwards and upwards with the same force
● if you sweep your arms to the right in aquafit, your whole body will move to the left; sweep them forwards and you'll move backwards …

And so it goes on, your limbs helping you to move in the desired direction by working them the opposite way.

### A little lift

What happens, therefore, if you stroke your hands inwards and outwards at a slight angle just under the surface? Sculling like this (see page 77) actually works on the same principle as a propeller, creating a downward pressure against the water to keep yourself at the surface. So sinker or no sinker, we can all learn to keep our heads above water, and enjoy more than a little 'lift' from our sessions in the pool.

# Part Two

# AQUAFIT

If you are a non-swimmer, make sure you are fully supervised at all times in the water, and that you practise the basic skills in Chapter 3 (see pages 20-22) before you start. You should also work out in waist-deep water rather than immersing yourself up to your chest.

# Chapter 4

# AQUACIRCUITS
## The Whole-body Workout

'Exercise should be pleasurable, not only as an incentive to do it, but because pleasure is good for us … Human nature being what it is, we will only continue to exercise if we enjoy it and feel that we are getting some benefit from it too.'

Glenda Baum, *Aquarobics*

Aquafit is a laugh – and a laugh which does you good. Where else can you lose your inhibitions while your body is fully supported and safe from injury? Where else can you avoid the threat of mirrors, and hide size, shape and lack of coordination? What else naturally balances your body up, works heart and lungs, muscles and joints? And what else can challenge, exhilarate, then perfectly relax you – and still get results? In short, what other workout is truly holistic?

## Aquacircuits

Nothing beats getting in there, getting wet, and following a qualified instructor to learn good technique, and there are obvious constraints once you try to translate this into book form, where you must visualize all the exercises and remember all the options.

Therefore, *Taking the Plunge* presents an easy-to-follow aquacircuit, including guidelines on adapting the moves to meet your individual needs. With no fancy choreography or complicated step patterns, it moves you smoothly from warm-up and pre-aerobic stretch to full circuits, cool-down and flexibility sections. It's designed to raise your heart rate and strengthen and stretch your muscles – and it works.

## Hold On!

Before we start, however, here are a few tips on posture and different ways of holding on to the side of the pool so that nothing interrupts your flow.

### Posture-check

If you go to any form of aerobics class nowadays, the first thing your instructor should do is a posture check to make sure that you stand in an easy, balanced position from which you can work safely and effectively – the idea being to try to align your ear, tip of the shoulder, hip-bone, knee and ankle if you look at

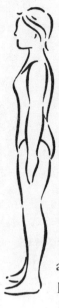

yourself side-on in a mirror. In other words, you want to flatten out the inward curve of the spine so as to 'protect' the lower back.

So before getting wet, stand with your back against the edge of a door, making sure your feet are about hip-width apart, your knees slightly bent – that is, not locked back tightly – and upper body lifted and relaxed. Now contract your abdominal muscles and tilt your pelvis so that your back doesn't feel over-arched. Test this by trying to slip your hand between your lower back and the door. If you can, contract those abdominal muscles a bit more and adjust your lower back a little.

Now try it in front of a mirror, turning to the side to watch the alignment of your body.

## Forward stance

However, a slight variation of this is needed to give stability to some movements. So, keeping your upper body in exactly the same position – neck and shoulders relaxed, chest lifted, stomach in and lower back flat through adjusting the position of your pelvis – change your footing so that one foot is a little in front of the other, still keeping your feet about hip-width apart, and your knees slightly bent. And when

you check your posture in the mirror again your body should still be centred, rather than leaning forwards, backwards or to either side.

When you're happy with both of these postures, practise them in the pool before trying the bracket hold.

## Bracket hold

Holding on to the edge of the pool with one hand, place the other, palm flat against the side and fingers pointing down to the floor, about a foot directly below it. Now pull on the top hand and gently push with the bottom, allowing your spine to straighten out and your feet to float out behind you.

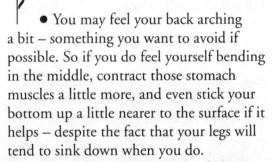

• You may feel your back arching a bit – something you want to avoid if possible. So if you do feel yourself bending in the middle, contract those stomach muscles a little more, and even stick your bottom up a little nearer to the surface if it helps – despite the fact that your legs will tend to sink down when you do.

• And eyes down! You may also feel an awkwardness in the neck area – bending it backwards as you try to look straight ahead. So if you *look down* into the water, with your face fairly close to the surface, this will bring your neck back into alignment with the rest of your spine.

Experiment with this hold until you feel quite comfortable with it, and take care of your wrists, neck and back.

You're now ready to begin.

# Chapter 5

# THE WARM-UP
## A Gentle Build-up

It's time for action, a gentle 10-minute warm-up to prepare both body and mind for the aerobic and muscular exercises in the main circuit.

---

Time invested in this part of your workout will pay good dividends.

---

● You want to work your way around your body, mobilizing each joint so that they move smoothly and safely. Try to act normally in the water. Move in a controlled and graceful manner, without cutting corners or becoming instantly uncoordinated.

● You want to raise your HR so that you steadily increase the flow of oxygen-rich blood around the body. Start slowly and build up gradually. Imagine you are in an elasticated tube – your arm and leg movements close to your body until you slowly ease off the restriction and the size of your actions increases. This is just an appetizer for what's to come.

● You want to make sure your muscles are nice and warm, increasing their elasticity so that they can work from full extension to full contraction.

● And you should gently stretch out your major muscle groups before beginning the circuit proper, to make sure they are firing on all cylinders!

Hygiene is not the only reason you should take a long hot shower before you start, because staying in there for a few minutes before getting into the water could actually start the process of warming up and increase your flexibility.

Each movement throughout the whole workout will be given in its simplest form to begin with, followed by a series of one or more progressions for the more advanced participant. If it's the first time you've done any aquatic exercise, though, take it easy to begin with, no matter what your level of fitness, and build up only gradually.

# The Build-up

Time: 10 minutes-plus, with at least a minute spent on each movement. Make sure that your HR is normal before you start and that you have topped up your system with fluid.

## Pulsing on the spot

A great name for a movement which begins the job of raising your HR so that your blood starts flowing around your body more quickly.

Stand feet hip-width apart in chest-deep water and by the pool edge to begin with. Bend your right knee so that the right heel is lifted and your weight is over on the left. Now simply shift your weight over to the right and back again, pulsing gently from side to side and allowing your arms to move as if you were walking along the road – right hand forwards as left heel lifts; left hand forwards as right heel lifts.

● Keep the supporting foot flat on the floor each side and the knee slightly bent.
● Always keep the big toe of the lifted foot in contact with the pool floor.
● Keep your upper body lifted and relaxed, shoulders down and stomach in.
● Breathe evenly.

## Progressions

● Add a slight bounce to the step, lifting up on to your toes a bit more but still staying on the spot. Make sure your feet land true, rolling from toes through to heels without your ankles falling inwards or turning out.
● Now lift your foot right off the floor each side, pumping your arms a little more vigorously now so that you are almost running on the spot. Again, think about how your feet strike the pool floor.
● And finally, allow your hips to sway gently from side to side so that you begin to mobilize your spine a little. Keep your upper body lifted and relaxed, with your shoulders square and stomach muscles tucked in.

## Water-walking

Again very simple, but surprisingly demanding when you want it to be. So hold fire until the circuits proper, and for now make use of water-walking's great warming and mobilizing potential. It also starts working on those under-used muscles in your backside and behind your thighs.

Walk forwards through waist- to chest-deep water for eight steps, and then go into reverse for eight, arms pumping and elbows bent. Repeat so that you get a feel for the movement.

Now concentrate on your feet again, rolling from heel through to toe as you walk forwards, and toe through to heel as you walk backwards. Repeat.

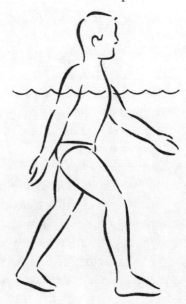

## Mobilizing your shoulders

Continue this but add some action in your upper body, first shrugging your shoulders up and down as you go, then rolling them in small circles forwards as you walk forwards and backwards as you walk back.

And finally make this action bigger by bringing your elbows into play, circling them forwards and back with your shoulders as you go.

● Watch your posture! Keep upright and lifted throughout, avoiding the temptation to lean forwards. Centre your head by looking in front of you all the time, keep your upper body relaxed and square and stomach muscles pulled in.

● Keep your lower back flat, especially when walking backwards. It's all too easy to arch it, so tuck those buttocks in.

● Almost exaggerate the foot action, flexing toe and heel on the forward and backward movements so that you begin warming up both the front of your shins and your calves.

● Don't hold your breath but keep your breathing even.

## Knee bends

With your pulse rate starting to rise a little now, start these stationary knee bends.

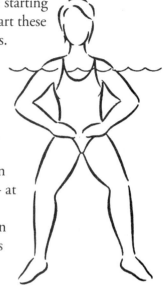

● Posture-check (see page 27). With your feet a little wider than hip-width apart and your knees and feet pointing outwards in the same direction – at about ten to two on the clock-face. When you bend your knees gently, they should travel out over your ankles.

● Never squat so low that there is less than a right-angle bend at your knees. (A mouthful of water may well remind you! )

---

# Trouble Spot

Many people suffer from knee problems, be it inflammation, pain when they walk downstairs, or as a result of some sort of injury. The knee is a complicated joint which needs looking after! Indeed, many people are encouraged to exercise in water if they have some kind of knee trouble because the pressure you place on them is drastically reduced when submerged. However, before doing a bit of DIY physiotherapy, check out any complaint you may have with a physio or at a sports clinic. Fitness is a specialized area, and your local doctor may not have experience in prescribing suitable exercises. And even if you don't suffer from any knee trouble, keep it that way with these three simple rules.

1. Always make sure that your knees point in the same direction as your feet so that they're never twisted or out of alignment.

2. Keep the joint just off the locked position.

3. Never twist the knee when you have your weight on it. And, of course, if it hurts – stop!

## Arm circles

Continue with your knee bends, but now add these upper-body movements to increase the mobility here. Begin where you left off in the water-walking with a few elbow circles before doing one full-arm circle forwards on each side, one full circle back as you gently bend your knees. (Good crawl practice!)

• Control the movements, especially as your arms break the surface. Keep the action slow and even so that the difference in resistance between water and air does not shock your muscles.

## Progression

• Repeat the full circles a maximum of four times each way – alternately on right and left, or in succession. It is a big movement, though, so watch that your pulse does not increase too quickly.

## Arm twists

Now, still doing gentle knee bends, hold your arms out in front of you and twist your hands back and forth at the wrists, warming up the base of the biceps muscles in your upper arms.

## Upper-arm action – 1

Now take the forward stance (see page 28) and bend your elbows, upper arms in at your sides and palms facing each other just under the surface so that they can slice through the water. Press alternate forearms down and up in a smooth chopping action to mobilize your elbows and warm up the opposing muscles in the upper arm – the biceps and triceps.

• Don't arch your back!

• Keep both hands under the water all the time.

• Always keep your elbows slightly bent, even when your hand reaches the bottom of the movement.

## Progressions

• Work both arms together rather than alternately.

• Alter the position of your wrists for more resistance, turning your palms upwards slightly as you press down and up. This is not a strength-training movement, though, just a warm-up, so don't push yourself too hard just yet.

## Knee lifts

It's time to pick up the lower-body action again with some simple knee lifts, taking alternate knees up to as near waist-height as is comfortable, with a two-footed bounce in the middle as you change legs. Hold on to the pool edge for balance to begin with, and once you're comfortable with the movement, pump your arms vigorously at your sides.

• Posture-check (see page 27)!

• Watch your landing, so that you roll down from toes to full foot on the bounce.

## Progressions
● Repeat the action four or eight times in succession on each side.
● Remove the middle bounce so that you increase the speed of your knee lifts – a bit like jogging with your knees up, so make sure you don't lean back.
● Travel forwards or to the right or left, again remembering that this is just a warm-up, not the circuits proper.

## Thigh presses
This is an excellent way of bringing your inner and outer thigh muscles into action.

Stand with your feet hip-width apart, feet and knees pointing outwards at ten to two on the clock-face. Shift your weight over on to your left foot and press your right heel – toes still out-turned – gently across in front of your left ankle. Jump as your feet come together again and repeat on the other side as your hands sway out the opposite way for balance.

● Lead with the side of your foot and your ankle.
● Keep your feet pointing outwards, or you won't work your inner and outer thighs.
● Keep your hips square to the front throughout the movement.

## Progressions
As with the knee lifts – travelling to the right as you press your right heel across and to the left as you press with your left.

## Space invaders
This continues working the inner and outer thighs but introducing a more intense upper-body movement for the deltoid muscles over your shoulders, as well as the pectorals and latissimus dorsi in your chest and back.

Keep your feet and knees pointing straight to the front this time as you take four steady side-steps to your right, four to

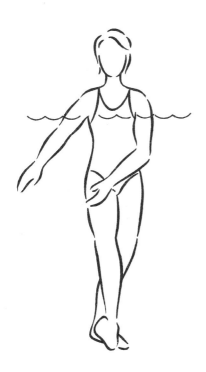

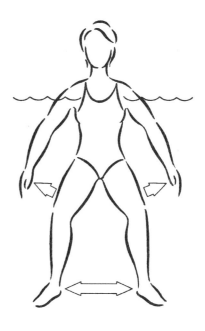

your left. Bend your elbows and on every step raise and lower them at your sides and back again chicken-style.

● Posture-check (see page 27)! Your neck and shoulders should be nice and relaxed and your stomach and buttocks tucked in.

● Bend your knees when you step out to the side, and keep them just off lock when they're together.

● Keep your hips square to the front, toes and knees pointing forwards.

● Breathe out as you step outwards, lifting your elbows.

## Progression

●Still leading with your elbows like a puppet, gradually straighten your arms until your elbows are just off lock, palms facing your thighs, keeping your neck relaxed at all times.

> ▲ When your arm is almost straightened, this move is very demanding – a strength-training exercise to be kept as an option for the circuit section of your workout. At this stage you're just warming up.

## The grind

And so to your lower back – crucial to remember, but easy to forget.

The grind is a small, controlled movement – basically a series of pelvic tilts to mobilize the lower back and begin warming up the abdominal muscles running down the centre of your stomach. To begin with at least, it's probably a good idea to stand at the pool edge with both hands on the side for support, knees soft, feet hip-width apart and upper body relaxed. Gently contract your stomach muscles so that your lower back curls inwards a little before releasing them again

as you return to your starting position. Repeat eight times, as long as you feel no discomfort. )

● Don't arch your back when you release the movement.

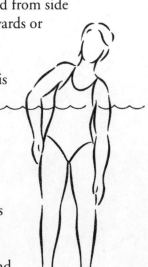

## Side bends

Side bends begin working on a different set of abdmonial muscles to the pelvic tilts – the so-called obliques wrapping around your torso – as well as mobilizing your spine.

Do a posture-check (see page 27), and then gently tilt your upper body a few inches to the right and then to the left so that your fingers slide up and down your thighs a couple of inches. Repeat eight times.

● Imagine that you are sandwiched between two boards. Bend from side to side, not forwards or back in any way.

● Keep it small. The movement is surprisingly restricted in its range of movement if done properly.

● Keep those stomach muscles contracted.

Now centre yourself again and from this position move smoothly into your pre-workout stretches.

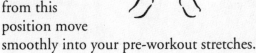

# Trouble Spot!

Statistically, you're in the very small minority if you don't experience some sort of back pain at some point in your life. There are many sources of trouble in this area, not least of which is muscular imbalance. This is not a physiotherapy guide and if you have back pain, seek medical advice. In the meantime, though, think about the following. Your spine can move in three planes. You can bend forwards and backwards at the waist; you can keep your hips square to the front and drop alternate shoulders so that you tilt your upper body to each side; and you can again keep those hips square and rotate your upper body gently at the waist.

Forwards and back, side to side and round and round. The three types of movement are quite distinct, and you can get into difficulty if you don't keep them this way – as when, for instance, bending down to one side to pick up a heavy suitcase. (Note that the oblique curls on page 59 are fine, however, since the movement is small and controlled, and your back fully supported.)

And remember that your spine includes your neck, so the wild neck-circling you often see at the gym is out! Again, think forwards and back, side to side and round and back.

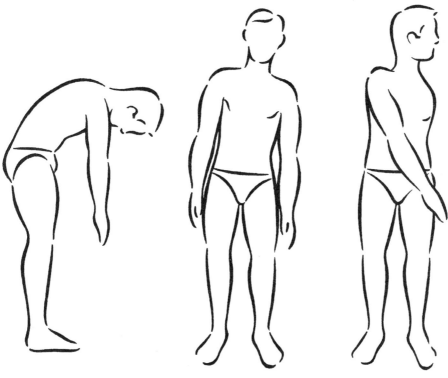

# The Pre-stretches

▲ Make sure your muscles are warm before you try to stretch them.

You'll find the information on stretching in Chapter 7 since the main flexibility section comes right at the end of your workout once your HR has started to drop and you've begun winding down.

Stretching should be productive, not destructive. Without allowing your body to cool down too much at this stage, you want to make sure that all the major muscle groups are at their full, working length before going into the aquacircuits proper. So spend about 10 seconds on each of the following (see pages 53–7): the chest and upper-back stretches; and both right and left sides for the hip stretch; the inner and outer thighs; the quadriceps stretch; the hamstrings stretch; and the two calf stretches – a total of nine in all.

# Chapter 6

# MAKING A SPLASH
## The Circuit to Results

'After the age of 20, a body loses approximately one pound of muscle every two years if no strength training is done …. For every pound of muscle lost, the metabolic rate goes down about 50 calories a day. For every pound of muscle gained, the metabolic rate goes up about 50 calories a day.'

Ruth Sova, *Aquatics*

And so to the main course, exercises which continue to raise your HR to a safe training level while strengthening and conditioning all the major muscle groups in your body. For ease of remembering, you'll work systematically from the bottom upwards – calves, thighs (front and back), hips, stomach (front and sides), arms, chest and shoulders – although once you're more familiar with the various components, you can obviously mix the upper- and lower-body exercises so as to work each group harder and for longer. Pace yourself for at least the first two or three workouts, though, because there's no point going mad at the beginning and having to give up halfway through, leaving some of your muscle groups untouched.

And the timing? This section can last for anything from 15 to 30 minutes, depending on your level of fitness. Start with a minute of each cardio exercise, and 30 seconds of each muscle, building this up over the coming months to two minutes on the cardios and one minute on the muscles.

▲ Stop an exercise if you feel any discomfort whatsoever, and use the 'pulse' at the start of the warm-up (see page 30) to keep the rest of your body moving. Go on to another exercise, or as with any workout, cool down and stretch out by following the guidelines in chapter 7.

Your HR should be just about approaching the lower end of your training zone when you start and finish this section, so check it quickly before you go any further. Make sure your system is topped up with water, and try not to push yourself too much on the muscles and spend the next cardio recovering.

## The Workout

Timing: 1–2 minutes for each cardio; 30 seconds to a minute on each muscle, depending on *you*.

## Cardio: water-walking

Begin your circuit as you began your warm-up – water-walking to increase your HR gently again after the more static pre-stretches. Walk forwards and backwards, gradually increasing the length of your strides as you go, and changing direction frequently.

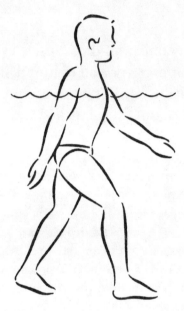

And the arms? Why not start off with a breast-stroke action as you move forwards, and an in-out pressing action at chest-height as you go backwards?

● Watch your posture! Keep upright and lifted throughout – avoiding the temptation to lean forwards. Centre your head by looking in front of you all the time, making sure your upper body is relaxed and square and stomach muscles pulled in.

● Keep your lower back flat, especially when walking backwards. It's all too easy to let it arch.

● Almost exaggerate the foot action, pulling those toes upwards as you move forwards so that you begin working on the

> For added intensity, change direction frequently. It's more difficult to repeat an action a few times in a lot of directions than it is to repeat it a lot of times in one direction.

muscles down the front of your shins again, and really lifting those heels on the way back, to focus on those calves.

● Keep your breathing regular.

## Muscle: heel and toe

This is a great way of continuing to work the lower leg – your shins and calves – while keeping your HR up so that you don't cool down.

> For all the muscle exercises, breathe out on exertion.

Supporting yourself side-on to the edge of the pool, repeat the knee lifts you did in the warm-up (see page 32) but this time doing four on each side *without the bounce in the middle*. Point your toes as your knee lifts, press down through the heel as it lowers again. Turn round and repeat on the other side, supporting yourself on the other side.

● Posture-check (see page 27)!

● Keep the knee of your supporting leg slightly bent.

● Concentrate on contracting the muscles in your shin as you point, those in your calf as you flex.

## Progressions

● Increase the number of reps on each side before changing – a maximum of 16.

● Increase the speed.

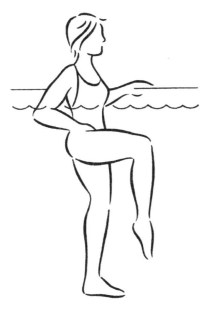
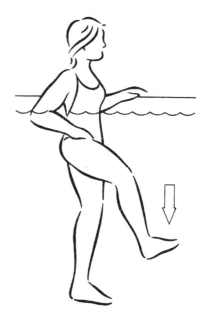

## Cardio: three-up jacks

An old favourite in aerobics classes, jumping jacks work the inner and outer thighs while raising the HR. However, as a slight variation on a theme, try the three-up jack for size.

Standing with your feet hip-width apart, toes and knees facing the front and lower back supported with strong abdominals, jump your feet apart into a wider stance. Jump them back again and then out once more, but this time bouncing once with your feet apart. In they come again, out, then in once more, and bounce, feet together; out, in, out and bounce and so on, your arms mirroring your leg action below the surface or out and up above the surface.

Water resistance increases with speed of movement. If you double the speed of your action, the resistance you'll have to work against goes up by four, giving you more propulsive force if swimming, and a more intense workout in aquafit.

- Watch your posture! Try to stay upright – not bending forwards or backwards at the waist.
- Keep your toes and knees pointing forwards, or at least in line with each other.
- Make sure your heels lower right to the pool floor, rather than bouncing away on your toes.

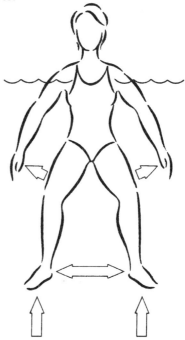

● Try to avoid breaking the surface with your arms as it is difficult to keep the action controlled. They should be raised and lowered below the surface, or lifted up and down above it.

## Progressions
● Increase the speed of your jacks.
● Increase the height of your jump.
● Travel! – either forwards, backwards or to either side. Pay special attention to your posture if you do, though, as it's all too easy to lean into the way you are moving.

## Muscle: curl kicks
And so to the front and back of your thighs – the quadriceps and hamstrings … and a perfect way to shape up.

---

To maintain good muscle balance, always work opposing groups evenly.

---

Holding on to the pool edge with your left hand, lift your right knee once more to about 45 degrees and support it with your right hand behind the thigh for stability. Draw your toes up towards your shin, and curl your foot back so that you bend your knee as far as is comfortable before kicking it forwards again to the starting position. Repeat four times on each side and change.
● Keep your thigh still throughout the movement so that only the lower part of your leg moves.

---

Feel the muscles behind your thigh work!

---

● Squeeze the muscles behind your thigh as you curl; contract the muscles at the front as you kick.
● Keep your hips square and upper body lifted throughout.

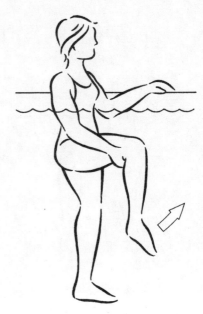

## Progressions
● Increase the number of reps each side, to a maximum of 16.
● Increase the speed.
● Relax your ankle so that your foot becomes floppy. You'll notice the increase in resistance immediately.

## Cardio: bouncing springs
With your feet apart and knees bent, spring forwards as far as you can, bouncing once on the spot when you've landed. Spring forwards again, and bounce again – springing and bouncing four times in a row forwards as your arms trace the breast-stroke action. Then repeat the pattern, springing and bouncing backwards, with your arms and cupped hands scooping forwards at your sides.
● This is a very demanding aerobic exercise, so take it easy to begin with.
● Posture-check (see page 27)! Use your arms to keep your body alignment true, trying not to lean forwards too much as you spring forwards, or backwards when you spring back.

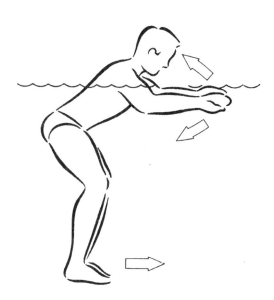

● Make sure you land properly, rolling down from toes through to heels, with feet and knees in line.

## Progressions
● Tuck your knees up underneath you as you spring forwards and backwards, pushing downwards more with your arms when they sweep back and forth to provide you with more lift.
● Increase the length of your springs and height of your bounces.
● Increase your speed.

▲ Pulse on the spot and check your HR. If it's too high – or if you can't hold a conversation easily or feel in any way uncomfortable – take it easy for a while. You can always be more energetic next time.

## Muscle: the lunge – with forward push
Moving on upwards, it's time to hit the buttocks and front of the thigh. The balancing arm action used will help you to maintain a good body alignment while also working your chest and upper back.

Stand with your feet hip-width apart and arms out to your sides with the palms facing the front. Gently shift your weight over on to your left foot and extend your right leg behind you until it touches the bottom with the ball of the foot. As you do so, draw your arms in front of you until your hands touch, before returning both top and bottom half to the start again. Repeat on the left.
● Contract those stomach muscles on the backward movement.
● Keep your weight forward when you extend your leg. (The arm action helps you do this.)
● Avoid pressing your heel down to the pool floor.
● Squeeze those buttocks when you step back; lead with the top of the thigh when you return to the start again.
● Control the movement – both in and out.

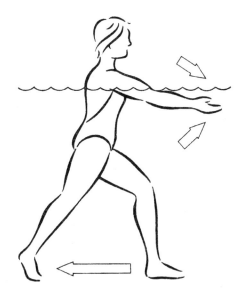

'Tone' is a slight tension in your muscles, giving them shape and definition.

## Progressions

- Repeat the action up to eight times in succession on each side.
- Increase the speed – without losing control.
- Increase the depth of your lunge and develop the return phase into a controlled knee lift, your arms again balancing the action by sweeping backwards slightly as your foot moves forwards. Hold those stomach muscles strong.

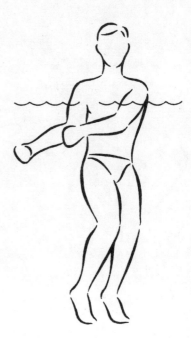

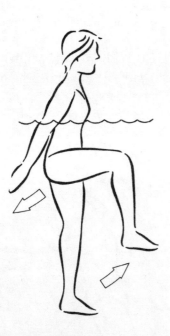

## Cardio: the skier

From a balanced starting position, bounce with both feet to right and left as if parallel skiing down a mountain, even drawing your hands backwards and forwards as if holding on to your poles.

## Progressions

- Keep your upper body fairly square to the front as your bottom half rotates from side to side if you wish to focus on your oblique muscles a bit more.
- Dig in, really bending your knees and springing upwards if it's your thighs you wish to work more.

## Muscle: side lift

And so to the inner and outer thighs, muscle groups which don't get worked very regularly in everyday life but which most people would like to see firmed up a bit.

Stand facing the pool edge, both hands extended for support. Your feet should be about hip-width apart as usual, and parallel. Keeping them this way, gently raise your right leg a few inches straight out to the side and lower it again, repeating with alternate legs.

- Posture-check (see page 27), making sure your stomach muscles are well contracted to support your lower back, and the knee of your standing leg slightly bent.

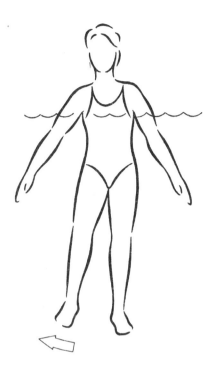

• Keep your toes, feet and hips square to the front. Turn them out to the side, and you work the hip flexors and buttocks again.
• Lead with the heel, pressing the outer thigh against the water to raise, squeezing inwards with the inner thigh to close.
• Keep the movement small and controlled.

## Progressions
• Do two, four or eight on the right before changing sides.
• Increase the speed.
• Curl your foot up towards your buttocks a little as you lift and lower, watching your posture all the time. (Below left.)

The greater the surface area you present to the water, the greater the resistance you'll encounter and the greater the intensity of the movement.

## Cardio: jogging on the spot
Pick those knees up, pump those arms and watch that HR rise! And to make it more demanding, travel forwards for eight steps, back for eight steps, punching out in front of you with alternate arms – even up over your head for added intensity.
• Watch your posture! Keep upright and lifted throughout, avoiding the temptation to lean forwards. Centre your head by looking forwards all the time, keeping your upper body relaxed and square and stomach muscles pulled in.

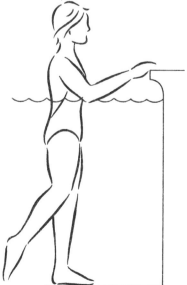

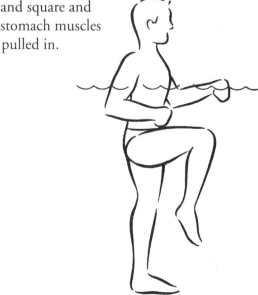

• Keep your lower back flat, especially when jogging backwards. It's all too easy to let it arch.

## Progressions
• Increase the length of your stride so that you bound through the water.
• Reduce the length of your stride, making the movement very quick and intense.
• Change direction frequently.

## The stomach
There are no two ways about it. The most important thing you need for safe and successful stomach work is stability – lying with knees bent, lower back pressed down into the ground and chin lifted as you focus on the central stomach muscle – the rectus abdominus – and the oblique muscles wrapping around your torso.

You obviously can't do this in a pool, though, so many aquafit classes try to incorporate abdominal work into their programmes in other ways. And there are various exercises you can try in which you work with your back to the edge of the pool, arms stretched out on either side to hold on and legs floating out in front of you as you attempt to curl your knees upwards and inwards towards your waist, or sweep both legs from side to side.

However, as soon as you try them you'll not only see how difficult it is to control the movements enough to squeeze those muscles properly, you may well feel some discomfort in your shoulders and particularly in your neck since it's virtually impossible to keep neck and spine in line when exercising in this position.

Therefore the aquacircuits are different. The stomach cruncher and side bends below will begin to work the major muscle groups in the abdomen, but for extra intensity and better results, try the three simple exercises in the Coda on page 58 as well – an added bonus to be worked at in the privacy of your own home.

## Muscle: stomach squeezer

Strong abdominals can help reduce the chance of lower-back problems through the added support they provide.

Standing with feet hip-width apart, do the grinding movement we used in the warm-up section to mobilize the lower back (see page 34), but this time up to 24 times in succession before resting for a moment or two. Hands resting on the top of your thighs for support, if you really squeeze your stomach in, you'll work that rectus abdominus from a good stable position.

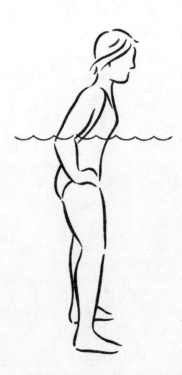

## Cardio: back kicks

A similar movement to the lunge with forward push on page 41, this movement also works the buttocks and hip flexors but with a small jump in the middle.

Kick your right leg backwards from the hip – knee straight – as your right arm punches forwards to compensate for the movement. Jump your feet together again and kick the left leg backwards, with the left arm punching forwards this time.
● Keep your stomach muscles well contracted, and neck and shoulders relaxed.

### Progressions

● Repeat the movement up to eight times in succession on each side.
● Bounce up higher in the water – while still watching your alignment!
● Remove the middle bounce so that the kicks follow one after the other.
● Travel backwards, being careful not to crash into anyone!

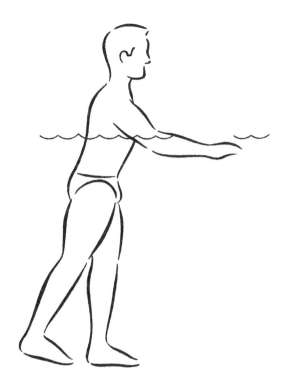

## Muscle: side bends

Repeat this exercise from the warm-up (see page 34), but up to 24 times in succession before pausing for a moment's breather. It is still a small, controlled action, though, so don't go mad just because we're in the conditioning part of the workout.

## Cardio: side raises – with downward press

Continuing the sideways theme, this is basically the same movement as the side lifts you did earlier (see page 42) but with a small jump in the middle – hopping alternate legs to the side with your toes pointing forwards, and bouncing with both feet together to change sides (see fig. 1 page 46). Indeed, you can even remove this

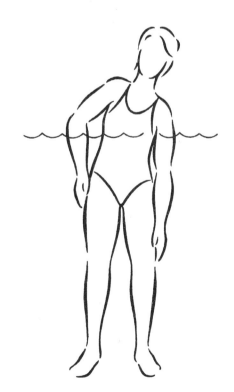

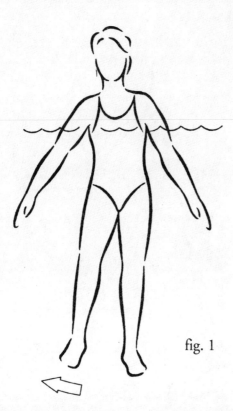

fig. 1

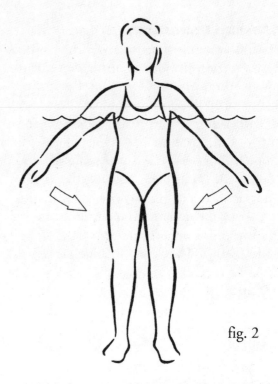

fig. 2

middle bounce entirely so that your legs sway smoothly from side to side. As before, concentrate on your body alignment so that you keep your stomach muscles strong and upper body lifted, and make sure you always lead with the edge of your feet, pressing inwards and outwards with your heels.

## Progression

● Add the downward press (see figs. 2 and 3). With arms raised out to the sides just below the surface – and with palms to the floor – squeeze downwards in front of you through the water with both arms as each leg is raised, really feeling that chest work. Then press your hands apart again to return to your starting position, this time focusing on the outer part of your shoulders. Keep your upper body well lifted throughout!

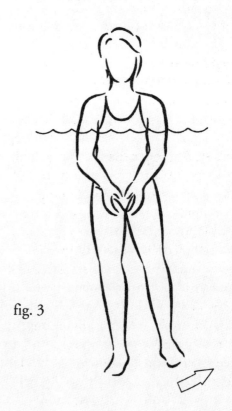

fig. 3

## Muscle: upper-arm action – 2

And now for the biceps and triceps – but doing the reverse of the upper-arm action in the warm-up.

From the forward stance (see page 28), knees slightly bent and stomach and buttocks tucked in, bend your elbows to about 90 degrees and draw them in to your sides. Now press them both backwards (hands facing down) until your wrists are level with your waist – elbows back about 4 or 5 inches (10 or 12.5 cm) behind you, chicken-style. Now press downwards and backwards with your hands until your elbows are almost straight, before returning to the starting position and repeating it about eight times before resting.

● Posture-check (see page 27)!
● Squeeze the back of your arms when you press back; the front of your arms when your press forwards again.

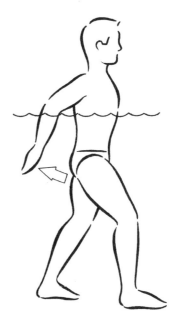

## Progressions

● Increase the number of reps.
● Increase the speed.
● Cup your hands as you press back.

## Cardio: tuck jumps

And so to the last of the really demanding aerobic exercises – the tuck jump to get you pumping.

From the standard starting position, arms out to each side, palms facing the bottom and just below the surface, press downwards firmly as you draw both knees up to your chest.

● Land carefully, rolling from the balls of your feet down into your heels.
● Keep your stomach muscles sucked in strongly.

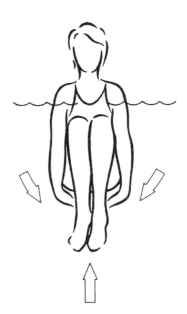

## Muscle: the squeeze-box

The second-last strength-training exercise works the chest and upper back. This time, make sure you are standing in slightly deeper water – up to your shoulders. Alternatively, bend your knees.

Stand square, feet hip-width apart,

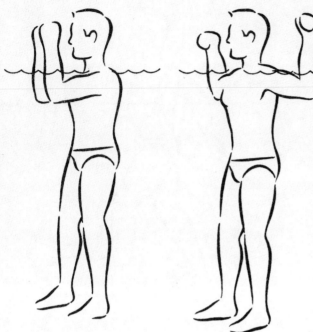

knees slightly bent, and tuck both stomach and buttocks under. Raise your arms as if in prayer, forearms and hands together and elbows lifted to about chest-height. Now draw them apart, pressing the arms outwards against the water before squeezing them back together again as far as is comfortable.

● Keep your upper body well lifted throughout.

● Make sure you don't arch your back when your arms are fully extended to each side. For extra stability, you might like to try this from the forward stance instead.

● Lead with your elbows when you draw them apart and back.

● Squeeze your chest muscles when your arms move inwards; your upper back when they return to the starting position.

## Progressions

● Increase the number of reps.

● Increase the speed and strength of the move.

## Cardio: rocking horse

This is a fairly gentle step working the hips, buttocks, lower back and abdominals. From the forward stance (see page 28), simply rock gently forwards and back so that you lift alternate feet a couple of inches off the bottom, your arms sweeping backwards as you move forwards and forwards as you shift your weight back again, to balance the movement. Repeat eight times before changing sides.

● Posture-check (see page 27)! It is essential that you keep your upper body completely flat throughout the movement, abdominals contracted to keep your spine from arching or bending.

● Try to keep your neck relaxed but still in line with your spine.

## Progressions

● Add a small hop as you rock forwards and backwards – sway–hop, sway–hop, and so forth.

● Rock your way around the pool.

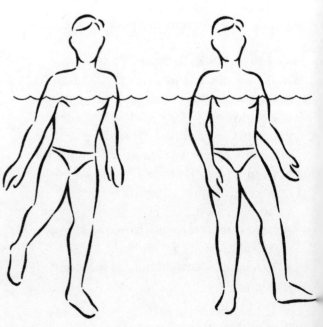

▲ Take your pulse again. It should be starting to come down a bit by now as you gradually begin to ease out of the circuit.

## Muscle: the U-swing

And finally to the deltoid muscles capping your shoulders – while working that chest and upper back a little more as well.

Feet slightly wider than hip-width apart, toes and knees pointing forwards, and arms at your sides, palms facing the front, slice your right hand through the water to your right while gently shifting your weight over to that side. Then, turning your palm inwards, slice your hand forwards until it's near the surface of the water. Draw it back down again, turn your palm to face the front once more and return it to the start as you centre yourself again to repeat the movement on your left – swinging it out and forwards, back and down, your hand slicing cleanly through the water as your body weight shifts to the left and back again. Repeat.

● Posture-check (see page 27)! And keep those abdominals well contracted.
● Keep your knees and feet in line, knees travelling over your toes as you sway to right and left.
● Keep your arms under the water throughout.

## Progressions

● Angle the position of your palms to increase the resistance, the back of the hand now leading as you push both to the sides and forwards.
● Sway both arms to right and left together.

● Lead with cupped hands for added resistance.
● Increase the speed of the movement.

## Cardio: water-walking – easing it out

See page 38 above, rolling your arms forwards and backwards as you move about the pool before simply pumping your arms gently by your sides.

Continue this last aerobic exercise for at least three minutes, gradually reducing the length of your steps, the vigour of your movements and your rate of your pulse.

It's time to start winding down, so continue with the gentle exercises and stretches in Chapter 7 before showering off once more.

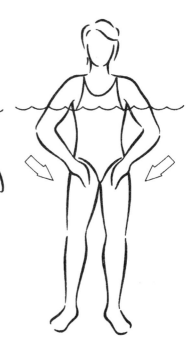

# WINDING DOWN AND STRETCHING OUT
## Cooling Off Your Workout

'By age 70, a person loses 20 to 30 per cent of his or her flexibility.'

Edward J. Shea, *Swimming for Seniors*

Just as you'd never change down from fifth gear to first when belting along in the fast lane, most people now know that coming to a grinding halt immediately after a vigorous workout is not such a good idea. Not only will the blood tend to collect in your legs, placing an unnecessary strain on your heart, you'll also prolong the time it takes your body to recover, not to mention encouraging muscular aches and imbalances in your body.

## Stretching Out

Flexibility is the one component of fitness that often misses the boat. It's essential to both the build-up and cool-down of any workout, and just because you feel more fluid when exercising in water, it doesn't mean you can cruise on past it in your

You are far less likely to ache after aquatic exercise than after land-based programmes because the amount of 'eccentric' muscle action is reduced (see page 23).

rush to hit the showers. Stretching out the major muscle groups after warming up ensures that they're firing on all cylinders when the real action starts, and when the workout's winding up and your HR down to normal, this also aids the body's recovery process – not only counteracting the muscle-shortening effect of exercise but beginning to disperse any lactic acid which can build up in the muscle tissue as well.

Age and immobility only go hand in hand if you let them.

So, as with every other component in the workout, there are dos and don'ts you have to remember when it comes to stretching out.

1. *Do* move into and out of position very gently.

2. *Do* breathe deeply and evenly, exhaling fully as you ease the muscles into the stretch. Your body will relax more.

3. *Do* only take the stretch as far as is comfortable – tension, but no pain.

4. And *do* maintain a good, balanced body alignment throughout.

But:

1. *Never* stretch out before your muscles are properly warmed up.

2. *Never* hold your breath.

3. *Never* bounce! The stretch should be even and steady, although in fact once the body is immersed the chances of bouncing are drastically reduced.

4. *Never* shake! If you feel your muscles twitching, ease out of the position a little.

5. And *never* be competitive. Just because the person next to you can tie themselves in knots, it doesn't mean you should try.

And which muscles should you stretch? Every one that has been worked. In other words, all the major muscle groups.

So even if you don't complete the full

---

'Maintenance' stretches last about 10 seconds, and are like on-going flexibility work, ensuring your muscles stay at their normal length. 'Developmental' stretches last at least 20 seconds, and do exactly as they say – *develop* or progressively lengthen a given muscle or muscle group which is normally tight for some reason.

---

circuit, or your muscles feel just pleasantly tired, do set aside a good 10 minutes at the end of your circuit to ease your body back to normality. And while in land-based exercise programmes the cool-down and flexibility sections are usually separated, in water you should keep moving gently in between stretches so that you don't let yourself get too cold.

# Winding Down

The following movements work systematically from top to bottom this time. The cool-down moves should last a minute each, with 10 seconds spent on each stretch. Exceptions are the hamstrings and inner thigh, which should be held for at least 20 seconds.

## Space invaders – arms bent

Repeat this movement from the warm-up (see page 33), but keeping the arm action small.

- Watch that body alignment!

## Shoulder stretch – 1

Continue side-stepping gently, but now add the first stretch – easing out all the tension around the back part of the shoulder. Without compromising your posture, and keeping your upper body and hips square to the front, draw your right arm diagonally across your torso and hold on to your wrist with your left hand, pulling it gently in towards your body. Repeat on your left.

- Relax your shoulders.
  - Keep breathing throughout the stretch.

### Shoulder stretch – 2

Now, still moving your lower body, ease out the shoulders around the sides.

Relax your neck, drop your left ear down towards your left shoulder a little, and this time draw your right arm behind you, gently pulling it across you again with your left. Repeat on the other side.

### Triceps stretch

And finally, reach up to the ceiling with your right hand, and drop it down between your shoulder-blades so that your elbow is still pointing straight upwards. Now gently ease that elbow backwards with your left hand by pressing on the underside of the right upper arm as it faces the front. Repeat on your left.

- Watch that posture! Keep your stomach and buttocks tucked well in so that you don't arch your back.
- Keep your neck and shoulders relaxed.

### Knee bends

Change the step now and return to some knee bends for a minute or so (see page 31). Gently sway your arms back and forth together by your sides, palms facing your sides.

- Make sure those knees and feet are pointing in the same direction!

### Upper back stretch

Now, with your lower body still ticking over, clasp your hands in front of you, drop your chin a fraction into your chest, and lift your arms up to the front, rounding your shoulders forwards so that your shoulder-blades ease apart behind you.

- Keep your buttocks tucked in.
- Make sure your elbows are slightly bent.
- Keep breathing!

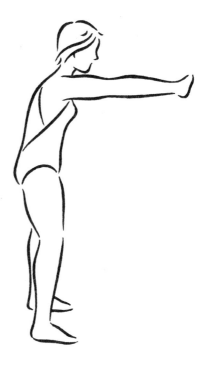

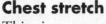

## Chest stretch

This time reverse the movement to stretch out your pectorals, biceps and the front part of your shoulder.

Clasp your hands behind you, elbows just off lock and squeezed together a little, and slowly lift your hands until you feel a gentle tension across your front.
● Don't arch your back accidentally, but keep those buttocks in.
● Lift your chest and drop your chin a little.
● And keep breathing evenly.

## The pulse

And onwards with the relaxed pulsing movement which began this whole workout. Gently pump the arms at your sides for balance, and try to bring that body twist into the action for a minute or so. Then stand with your feet hip-width apart, toes and knees pointing outwards slightly, knees just off lock and buttocks tucked under for the next two stretches to the abdominal muscles.

## Waist stretch

Keeping your hips square by placing your left hand on your left hip, lift your right arm up and very slightly over your head. Repeat on the other side.

● Lift upwards out of your pelvis.
● Stay upright, without bending forwards or back.
● Keep those buttocks in.
● Don't over-bend to your side.

## Stomach stretch

This stretch should be done very gently, because in order to release any tension in the rectus abdominus running down the centre of the stomach, you have to arch your back slightly – something you normally wish to avoid. SO TAKE CARE.

Centre yourself, and this time clasp your hands over your head so that you can still see them if you look up. Now, lift up your rib-cage and push your chest forwards a little until you feel a gentle tension down the front of your stomach.
● Keep your breathing steady.
● Relax your shoulders and neck.

## Space invaders

Return to a minute of side-stepping (see page 33), pumping your arms gently by your sides.

## Outer-thigh stretch

On one leg this time, bend your right knee and draw it upwards and across your body with both hands as far as is comfortable – almost as if you were crossing your legs if sitting down. Now ease it inwards towards your left shoulder until you feel a slight tension around the outer thigh. Repeat on your left.

● Keep your supporting knee slightly bent.

● Your upper body should be nice and relaxed, and lifted.

## Inner-thigh stretch

Changing sides again, lift your right knee once more, and this time, supporting it underneath with your right hand, draw it gently out to the right side until you feel the stretch on the inside of your thigh. Repeat on your left.

● Hold this stretch for at least 20 seconds.

● Keep your supporting knee slightly bent.

● Your upper body should be nice and relaxed, and lifted. Both these stretches release tension in the buttocks as well, so we won't be doing anything special with them on their own.

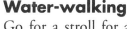

## Water-walking

Go for a stroll for a moment or two (see page 30), pumping your arms gently by your sides.

## Hamstring-stretch

Stand facing the edge of the pool and lift your right foot up as high as is comfortable so that the heel is flat against the side. Keeping your upper body lifted and square to the wall, lean forward slightly at the waist before gradually straightening your right knee until you feel a gentle tension down the back of the leg. Repeat on your left.

● Hold this stretch for at least 20 seconds.

● Keep your supporting knee slightly bent, with knees and toes pointing straight ahead.

● Make sure your upper body is lifted, pulling upwards and out of your pelvis when you lean forwards.

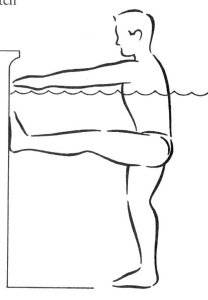

## Quadriceps stretch

Holding on to the side of the pool with your left hand, draw your right heel up towards your buttocks until you can hold on to your ankle with your right hand. Gently ease your heel back towards you until you feel some tension down the front of the thigh. Repeat on the left.

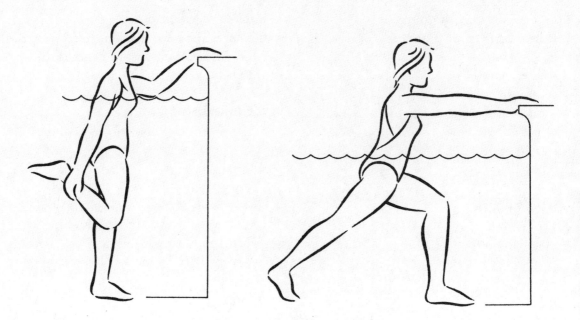

● Posture-check (see page 27)! Keep that lower back flat and stomach pulled in.

● Keep your thighs fairly close together, the bent knee pointing down to the floor – even behind you a little to begin easing out your hips.

● Your supporting knee should be slightly bent. You might find it more comfortable if you swap hands – your right hand holding your left foot, and your left hand your right foot.

## Hip stretch

And so to the muscles we use every time we walk, every time we go upstairs – muscles which we usually forget to look after. The quad stretch above already began releasing the tension in this area, and this one will do it even more.

In shallow water, go into the lunge position from the circuits (see page 41), your right leg forwards to begin with and holding on to the side of the pool for support. Now, with upper body lifted, and right knee over your right ankle, slide your left foot backwards on the toes as far as is comfortable. Then, to increase the stretch even more, straighten the left knee – but gently! Ease out of position and swap sides.

● Posture-check (see page 27)! Keep that stomach well contracted.

## The pulse

Pulse it out once more (see page 30), just lifting your heels off the pool floor this time in a gentle, relaxed action. Just the calves to go now!

## Calf stretch – 1

From the forward stance (see page 28), lean forwards from the hips so that your right knee is bent, supporting yourself with both hands about halfway down your right thigh. There should be a gentle diagonal running all the way up from your left heel to the top of your head.

● Make sure that your heels and toes are

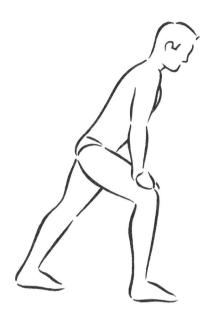

over your back heel, hands clasped loosely behind your buttocks. You should feel the stretch lower down in your ankle.

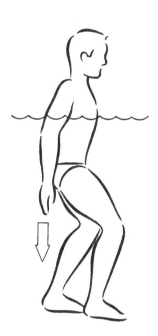

in line, both feet pointing straight to the front. So look downwards, particularly checking your back heel. If it is turned inwards, get it in line again. Indeed, if you're having problems even keeping it down in the water, imagine lifting your toes up on that foot.

● Check that the knee of your front leg is directly over your ankle – not pressed forwards over your toes.

● Keep your stomach muscles contracted and upper body relaxed, your head and neck in line.

● Keep breathing evenly.

## Calf stretch – 2

Now, from that position, draw your left foot in towards your right, and 'sit down'

● Tuck your buttocks in to keep your lower back flat.

● Make sure your toes and heels are in line.

● Keep your upper body relaxed.

Repeat both stretches on the other side.

And if you're not too cool by now, lie back into a relaxing float for a few moments (see page 20), eyes closed, chin and chest lifted, to ease away any last remnants of tension. You've worked hard. What's called for now is a nice hot shower.

# ABDOMINAL EXTRAS

The following three stomach exercises complement those in the aquacircuits and can be done in the privacy of your own home for that extra bit of toning.

## Stomach curl

Lie on your back, with knees bent and feet about hip-width apart and a comfortable distance from your backside. Raise your hands in front of you so that they rest gently on your thighs, about halfway between hip and knee, and now curl forwards carefully until your shoulders are no more than a couple of inches off the floor. Your hands should end up resting gently at knee-level. Return to your starting position and repeat eight times. Pause for a few moments, then do another set of eight curls.

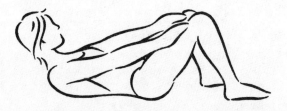

● Keep your lower back pressed down on to the floor at all times.
● Really squeeze those stomach muscles as you lift, and control the movement as you lower again.
● Imagine you've got an apple stuck under your chin so you keep it well lifted throughout the movement – eyes raised and looking upwards towards the ceiling in front of you.
● Keep the movement smooth, controlled and small. Wrenching your shoulders forwards will use momentum to curl you upwards rather than focusing on your stomach.
● Breathe *out* as you curl forwards, and in again as you slowly return to your starting position.
● And never anchor your feet underneath anything. If you do, all the work will be done by your hip flexors, not your stomach.

## Progressions

● Increase the number of sets.
● Slow the speed of your curls.
● Cross your arms over your chest.
● Rest the tips of your fingers at your temples, elbows pointing straight out to each side, and chin lifted. The movement should still be small and controlled, focusing on the abdominal muscles.

▲ Never cup your hands behind your head or neck and jerk your shoulders off the floor.

## Stomach cruncher

This exercise is basically the same as the stomach curl above except that your feet are raised off the floor – a good right-angle bend at both hip and knee.

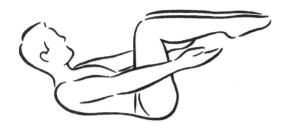

Indeed, you can even practise this with your heels resting gently on top of a stool to make sure you have the correct position. This will also allow you to concentrate more on squeezing those abdominal muscles tight as you slowly lift those shoulders a couple of inches off the floor.

## Progressions

As for the stomach curl above.

## Oblique curl

And finally, to shape up that waist a bit more, here's another simple adaptation of the stomach curl above.

This time you gently twist at the start of the movement so that your right hand reaches across your body and over to your left knee before returning to your starting position.

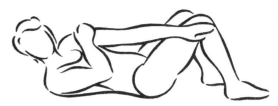

● Keep your left shoulder firmly planted on the floor throughout the movement.

Repeat eight times and swap sides, your right shoulder glued to the floor this time as your left hand reaches across to your right knee.

## Progressions

● Increase the number of sets.
● Reduce the speed of your curls.
● Rest the tips of your fingers at the temple of your twisting side, elbow pointing straight out as with the stomach curl above.

And now slowly ease out by rolling gently on to your front and lifting yourself up on to your elbows for about 10 seconds while looking downwards to keep your neck and back in good alignment. You're on your way to a strong and well-toned stomach.

▲ If you're pregnant avoid abdominal exercises lying on your back like this after the fourth month.

**Chapter 8**

# AQUANATAL
## The Active Pregnancy

'We live in water for the first nine months of our lives ... the constant caress of water on our skins gives us our very first sensations ... [and] help to give us our first primitive sense of 'self', of who we are, of where we begin and end ... The birth of a child follows the breaking of the water and the opening of the womb.'

Janet Balaskas and Yehudi Gordon, *Water Birth*

Water and babies have a natural association. It was a Soviet swimming instructor, Igor Tjarkovsky, who first pioneered the idea of underwater births in the 1960s, and the subsequent work of Dr Michel Odent at the maternity unit in Pithiviers, France, has been enormously important in giving women more control over the type of delivery they have. Extreme this approach may be. Nevertheless, a gentle aquafit class at the local pool is often the first port of call for women interested in having an active pregnancy, recognising almost instinctively that while actually giving birth in water is not for them, this is the ideal medium for an antenatal fitness programme.

● Your movements are slowed, allowing you more time to react if you lose your footing, and giving you an added sense of security through the support it offers – especially as full term approaches

● You feel relaxed and refreshed as the water massages you from top to toe, easing away discomfort in your back and lower body as gravity loses its force against the upward lift of buoyancy.

● And more than anything else, you feel light and graceful when on dry land you can feel all too heavy and clumsy

To look at exercise during pregnancy in any detail would be a book in itself, and if you are pregnant or thinking about starting a family, the chances are that you have already bought up all the material on nutrition, health care and parenting you can find so as to supplement the guidance offered by your doctor. It would be unrealistic, therefore, to try to do more than whet your appetite in a short chapter like this, introducing you to a few of the most basic ideas and providing some general pointers about what to look for in a good aquanatal class. If you want to find out more, the books highlighted in the list of Suggested Reading on page 128 – and particularly the Melpomene Institute's *Bodywise Woman* – come highly recommended.

▲ KEEP YOUR DOCTOR INFORMED. Discuss your plans to exercise before getting your feet wet – especially if there is some medical condition which might affect you or your pregnancy. Once following a recognised aquanatal programme, let your doctor know how you are getting on, checking with them if you have any questions, or if your pregnancy changes for any reason – like discovering you're having twins, for instance. And stop exercising immediately if you have any pain, nausea or vomitting, excessive breathlessness or elevated HR well after the aerobic workout has finished, dizziness or lack of co-ordination, or prolonged fatigue. Exercise is a two-way process: it's not just about training your body to cope with new challenges in the future, but learning to listen to it and being flexible in your approach.

# The Active

Don't push yourself to prove that nothing has changed. Do what feels good, and be cautious with physically demanding activities that you have not done before.
Femmy DeLyser, *Jane Fonda's New Pregnancy Workout and Total Birth Program*

# Pregnancy

In many ways, the aquanatal workout is no

If you haven't exercised for some time before getting pregnant, spend the first trimester getting used to all your body's changes, and only then add a gentle but regular workout to your diary.

bility and relaxation covered in the preceeding chapters – albeit to a greater or lesser extent. A good class, however, will also include a period at the end where you can ask questions and swap experiences with the other members of the group, and this often offers you the chance to spend a bit of time with your instructor as well, modifying your workout to meet your individual needs and discussing alternative exercises. After all, no two women are the same – let alone two pregnancies.

● Wear either a comfortable maternity swimsuit with inner protection for your breasts, or a sports bra under your normal costume.

● Stay cool! Avoid working out in hot and humid conditions, and take extra care to drink lots of fluid before and throughout the class. Similarly, avoid saunas and hot tubs (see page 118) for the first few months, and if you do fancy a steam after that point, keep the temperature down and the length of time short – less than 15 minutes.

● Take care when walking along the poolside to avoid slipping, and always enter the water by the steps rather than jumping in feet first or diving. Turn round and descend backwards one step at a time if the steps are vertical, and make sure you support yourself with both hands.

● Exercise in shoulder-deep water if possible so as to benefit from all the support and buoyancy it offers. However, if you haven't become confident in the pool yet, keep the water at waist-height or stay near the edge, holding on whenever necessary.

## Posture-check

Good body alignment is important whenever you exercise, but during pregnancy your COG changes as the baby grows, and it's all too easy to compensate for this by allowing your lower back to arch and shoulders to slump forwards – adding to the chances of backache and strain to the backs of the legs. The posture-check here is no different from that on page 27, although do pay particular attention to the following.

● Keep your body centred over your feet, and knees just off lock.

● Tuck your pelvis forwards and think about taking the baby backwards towards your spine, concentrating on flattening out the inward curve of your lower back.

● Focus on your upper body, lifting upwards from your hips, with your neck and spine in line, and shoulders relaxed but pulled back a little.

## Deep breathing

Indeed, modifying this stance slightly gives you an excellent position in which to practise deep and regular breathing.

Standing in the shallow end, with your back to the poolside and your feet parallel and about hip-width apart, bend your knees into an easy squat so that your shoulders are just above the surface. Rest your back against the pool wall and as before, flatten it out by tilting the base of your pelvis forward, this time lengthening your spine by allowing your chin to drop gently towards your chest. Cradle your

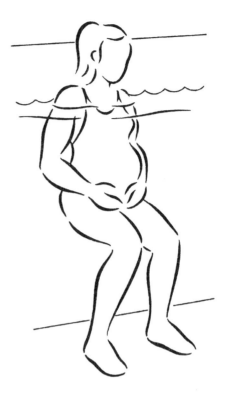

baby with both hands under your stomach, and close your eyes, focusing on exhaling fully through your mouth and inhaling through your nose.

# The Warm-up

Because you want to ease your body very gradually into the workout ahead, spend an extra two or three minutes on this part, taking at least 12 minutes to warm up (see pages 29–36). Focus more on mobilizing movements and upper-body work than on leg actions which raise your breathing and heart rate excessively. Take it easy, incorporating the following exercises aimed specifically at working your lower back and thighs, as well as releasing tension and improving mobility in the pelvic area.

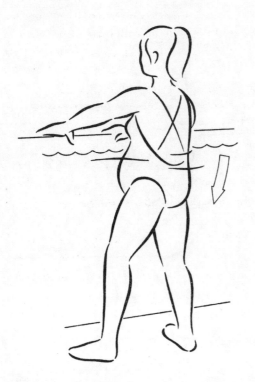

• Make sure your knees and feet are pointing in the same direction.
• Make sure your back is flat and upper body relaxed when you release the tuck. Arching is out!
• Keep your breathing steady and deep throughout.

## The belly dancer

A wonderfully sensual movement. Draw your feet closer together until they are about hip-width apart, toes pointing straight ahead of you and knees just off lock. Flatten out your back and gently gyrate, circling your hips 10 times to the right, 10 times to your left.
• Keep your upper body lifted and relaxed.
• Make sure your knees and feet are pointing in the same direction.
• Try not to arch your back too much as you rotate.
• Keep your breathing steady and deep throughout.

## The slow grind

Similar to the exercise on page 34, the slow grind helps your posture by rounding the base of your spine, as well as gently mobilizing the abdominal muscles.

Facing the side in waist-deep water, move your feet fairly wide apart, bend your knees and hold on to the edge of the pool with both hands for support. Staying in that position, now tilt your pelvis forwards as if exaggerating the posture-check and hold this position for a second or two before releasing slowly. Repeat the movement 8 times.

There are about 36 pairs of muscles attached to your pelvic region, making it the focal point of your lower abdomen and upper thighs – and as you know, crucial in childbirth.

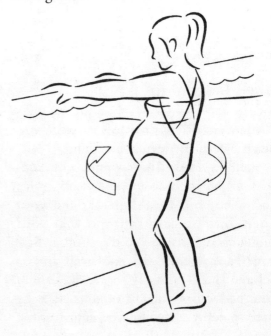

As in Chapter 5, stretch out all the major muscle groups before continuing with your workout (see also page 66 below).

# Strengthening Exercise

As in the warm-up, aquanatal workouts often give prominence to movements which gently condition the muscles in the stomach and lower back, and the stomach squeezer on page 34 is a good option, as are the side bends which bring the oblique muscles criss-crossing your stomach into play. However, there's nothing to stop you practising your pelvic-floor exercises in the pool as well, helping to safeguard against problems at birth, and improving your recovery rate afterwards.

▲ Avoid abdominal exercises like those on pages 58–9 after the fourth month since lying on your back to work them is not recommended. And check with your doctor if you feel the muscle running down the centre of your stomach separating by more than a couple of fingers'-width.

Don't forget your top half. Good muscle tone in your upper back will not only benefit your posture but, in conjunction with a few exercises for your chest and arms, will also pay dividends in the future by preparing you for carrying your baby around. Try the upper-arm action on either page 32 or page 47, the squeeze box on page 47 and the U-swing on page 49, keeping your body aligned and balanced throughout, and the number of repetitions fairly low.

Water has about 12 times the resistance of air, naturally improving general muscular conditioning while keeping your body fully supported (see page 22).

# Aerobic Workout

While it might not feel it at the time, you're actually at the peak of aerobic fitness during pregnancy. Moderate exercise during these nine months is comparable to vigorous exercise at other times, but there are a few things to bear in mind. Because your HR is higher than normal, and you not only need to keep your core temperature down but a good supply of blood to your baby the whole time, the American College of Obstetricians and Gynecologists (ACOG) recommends that this section lasts a maximum of 15 minutes and that you monitor your HR carefully, making sure that it stays below 140 bpm the whole time.

Your body may well tell you to do this naturally, though, since an increased sensitivity to $CO_2$ will make you feel more breathless than normal anyway. Stick to no-impact movements like gentle knee bends (see page 31) – always concentrating on good body alignment and keeping your pelvis tucked under – not to mention low-

Make sure that you eat enough to meet not only the extra energy demands of being pregnant, but your aquatic workout as well.

A regular 20-minute immersion has been shown to be very effective against pregnancy edema – or the swelling many women suffer from in the ankles and feet.

impact steps like water-walking (see page 30) and space invaders (see page 33), pressing the water aside as you go rather than suc-cumbing to the temptation to bounce. After all, working the large muscle groups in the lower body like this has the added benefit of improving your circulation, as the muscles squeeze against the veins running up the legs and help pump the blood back up to the heart.

# Cool-down and Flexibility

As with the warm-up, don't cut short this part of your workout in your rush to hit the showers. Instead, spend an extra couple of minutes building out of the aerobic section (about 12 minutes in all) so that your HR gradually returns to a more normal level. However, when stretching out as the class comes to a close (see chapter 7), the opposite approach applies. Hold your stretches for a shorter length of time (about 6 seconds each) so that your major muscle groups simply return to their resting length rather than trying to increase their range of movement in any way. One of the many changes that takes place during pregnancy is a softening of the ligaments caused by the release of a hormone called, appropriately enough, relaxin. And while this is really designed to loosen up the

pelvic region to ease delivery, its action also affects all your other joints, which can become unstable and more prone to injury. Needless to say, avoid all bouncing movements when holding a stretch.

# Relaxation

Finally, find a quiet part of the pool and pause for a moment or two, breathing deeply and feeling any last touches of tension drain away as your weightless body floats in the soothing, refreshing water.

# Aquanatal Exercise

You should begin improving your level of fitness before becoming pregnant, of course. And if nothing else, this momentous time in your life could be all the inspiration you need to take the plunge in the first place – the natural desire to see your body return to more normal dimensions after the birth being all it takes to progress from a gentle postnatal workout into a more demanding programme.

For those of you already exercising two or three times a week, however, you should be able to carry on with your normal programme for a few months, letting your

Reportedly, three gold medal winners in the 1956 Olympics (Melbourne) were pregnant...and in 1952 a pregnant diver won third place.

Christine L. Wells, *Women, Sport and Performance*

three times a week, however, you should be able to carry on with your normal programme for a few months, letting your body tell you how and when to ease off. For instance, if following either of the swimming programmes in Chapter 13, use this time to focus on your technique rather than distance, stopping any interval training (see page 112) until well after the birth so as to keep your HR and temperature down (see pages 62 and 65 above).

---

Aim to *maintain* your level of fitness rather than improve it during pregnancy.

---

Vary your strokes as much as possible, working all the major muscle groups and changing swimming style if you feel any leg cramps or joint pain. Pay particular attention to keeping your head and neck in line when swimming on your front, and concentrate on breathing properly throughout your swim so as to keep an even supply of oxygen to both your own body and your baby's. Sculling is relaxing yet strengthening (see page 77), and as your pregnany progresses, you might find side stroke more comfortable than floating on your back.

Whatever your level of fitness, though, you should feel refreshed and invigorated at the end of your workout, the exercise giving you energy rather than sapping you of strength. Remember: exercise is only one of many variables which can affect the outcome of your pregnancy, and every woman is different. So find out as much as you can, choose your classes carefully, and enjoy the sense of freedom that a water workout can bring. The right workout at the right time can be both physically satisfying and emotionally fulfilling as you take an active involvement in your own and your child's well-being. And brief though this chapter is, it has hopefully inspired you to think a little more about the opportunity of aquatic exercise during pregnancy.

## Part Three

# SWIMMING

# Chapter 9

# TAKE A DEEP BREATH . . .
## Basic Skills with a Touch of Inspiration

For well over 2000 years, the shellfish and edible seaweed along the stunning shores of Korea and southern Japan have been the inspiration for what has to be one of the most outstanding feats of human endeavour. And it's a feat still repeated for several hours a day, year in and year out, by some 10,000 women aged between 11 and 65. With nothing more than a face-mask and in some cases weights to help them go down, the *ama*, or diving women, descend to depths of between 60 and 80 feet to harvest their crops, holding their breath for nearly two minutes at a time and in temperatures as low as 10°C. All this with only a few moments' rest between dives.

> Even in water above 20°C you can get hypothermia if exposed for long enough. And below 15°C, untrained people can normally only hold their breath for a maximum of 15–25 seconds.

Of course, it would be nice to be able to draw some conclusion about the superior endurance and breath-holding ability of the female sex when talking about the *ama*, but in fact neither women nor men hold a marked advantage here. The hist-orical explanation for why the *amas'* work has been taken on by women is apparently that from the 6th century onwards army conscription in these countries prevented men from following this underwater way of life, although local folklore has a more interesting reason: the taste sea-bream acquired for men's testicles.

So are the *ama* special? The answer has got to be yes, simply because of the way they train their bodies to cope with this incredible diving lifestyle – seeking the depths from an early age right up to the delivery of the next generation and nursing

> At the sort of depths *ama* dive to, you're looking at a pressure of 2–3 tons per square foot working against the sensitive membranes of the inner ear, and compressing the air in the lungs to *half its normal volume.*

the baby in the boat between diving shifts. Not that this is recommended, of course.

*Ama* means 'ocean' or 'air' in Old Japanese.

But as to whether or not the *ama* could be genetically predisposed to this kind of breath-holding ability, the answer seems to be no. And the somewhat surprising conclusion must be that you or I could well have been *ama*, had we trained in the right way. For much closer to home, women are undertaking incredible feats of breath-holding, strength and flexibility every day, remaining submerged for up to a minute and half at a time and in up to 10 feet (3 metres) of water: they are the much maligned synchronized swimmers.

# The Desire to Breathe

The first thing to remember about breathing is that it isn't a lack of oxygen in the lungs which causes you to take the next breath but the build-up of the waste product carbon dioxide ($CO_2$) in your blood. On dry land, of course, you rarely even think about breathing unless you have some kind of respiratory disorder like asthma. However, once in the water you have to inhale and exhale *consciously,* coordinating your breathing with your strokes so that you become acutely aware of the 'breaking-point stimulus' which forces you to draw air into your lungs.

Swimming has been shown to be beneficial to asthma sufferers, helping them learn to control the frequency of their breathing.

With training, the body can adjust to higher levels of $CO_2$ in the blood, and you can even achieve a slight build-up effect over the period of a few minutes. Indeed, one test demonstrated that breath-holding times could be increased by as much as 25–30 per cent over six attempts in quick succession. It's an interesting fact to remember if you are still anxious about the prospect of going underwater – although obviously breath-holding on its own like this is definitely not to be recommended. And on top of that, breath-holding swimmers actually improve their ability to tolerate lower levels of oxygen in the blood as well (hypoxia). Indeed, top-level synchro swimmers train with 'unders and overs', swimming a length of a given stroke above water, followed by another length of it submerged, 12 times in succession and with only a few seconds' break at each end. And while the space occupied by the lungs in the rib-cage can't grow any bigger,

> Tricks of the trade: allegedly you can also enhance your breath-holding ability through swallowing, forced expiration or gently poking yourself in the eye – reflexes commonly used to diagnose various medical conditions. Not that anyone would recommend using any of these in the water, though!

swimming training does increase their volume by using this limited space more efficiently, increasing your so-called 'vital capacity' so that, quite simply, you can take a deeper breath.

There's one last factor to consider when it comes to breath-holding, though – a complex set of reflex responses which inspire tearful close-ups in *Baywatch* and make headline news when 'drowned' people are brought back to life...

# The Diving Response

People can be revived up to half an hour after 'drowning' in cold water.

Under normal circumstances your blood delivers oxygen and nutrients to every part of your body while simultaneously removing any waste products – $CO_2$ included. However, if you are unable to breathe for any reason, your body has to conserve its oxygen stocks: exactly what happens when the so-called 'diving response' is stimulated. Slowing the HR and changing the distribution of circulating blood, it channels the flow away from the arms and legs – which can survive without it for about half an hour – and redirects it towards the brain and heart, vital organs which suffer critical damage after just a few short minutes of oxygen deprivation. It's a response triggered by simple breath-holding, but intensified during immersion by special and little-known areas detecting water around our eyes, nose and neck, and it's dramatically increased if the water is cold – especially if you exercise at the same time. Indeed, this last factor is possibly another reason why we have a lower HR during aquatic exercise than when working out on dry land.

So what does all this mean for our appreciation of the skilful demands of synchronized swimming?

# 'Underwater basket-weaving' and 'Synchronized drowning'?

Lying upon his back straight as before, his hands with their palms downwards, pressing the water the better to keep him up, he must cast both legs out of the water at once, and caper with them upwards as men oft to do downwards in dancing...
Everard Digby, *The Art of Swimming*, 1587

When it comes to swimming and water agility, little has really changed over the last four centuries, it seems, although nowadays synchronized swimming gets bad press. It's worth considering why for a moment. David Pratt's review of the 1992 Olympic coverage in the *Daily Mirror*, for example, referred to it as 'comic relief' and 'a popular distraction from the otherwise serious business', and his views reflect the age-old argument about what does, and

> We are starting to see some returns to 'heavier costuming'. Is it necessary? Is it desirable? Is it appropriate for sport? Do we need rules to curb this dangerous trend?
>
> Judith McGowan, *The Past, the Present, and the Future of Synchronised Swimming as a Sport*, 1993

what does not, constitute a 'sport', and whether or not artistic impression has a valid place in the Games. If he'd applied such dismissive attitudes to the ever-popular gymnasts, however, or the crowd-pulling figure-skaters or competitive divers, there would have been uproar. None of these events can be won 'objectively' because as with synchro, they are all dependent on a subjective assessment of execution and artistic impression.

It seems that here, as everywhere else in life, dual standards come into play. Such standards condemn displays of supreme athleticism in synchro swimmers while allowing the inclusion of the likes of rifle-shooting because of its association with hunting and manly achievement. Or maybe it's more to do with the fact that it's an exclusively female sport?

Nevertheless, it's easy to see why people tend to smirk at the mention of synchro. The sparkling costumes – currently under debate with the ASA Synchronized Swimming Committee – are an obvious target and one which could well take a nose-dive in the near future. Then there are those frantic-looking arm movements and theatrical poses – acceptable in gymnastics, it seems, yet mocked if performed in water. But who stops to think about the sheer power needed in the lower body to hold the swimmers not only steady in the water but elevated up to their waists above the surface (and without the help of the foam-filled belts currently gaining popularity in aquafit workouts)? Or the incredible arm and hand control necessary to allow the legs to remain elevated in a certain position or emerge gracefully from the depths before sinking slowly back under again?

> During a figure like the heron, the raised leg weighs an enormous amount in comparison with the seeming weightlessness of the rest of the body.

Indeed, viewing from the safety of an armchair, we get no sense of scale, no feel for how big an area of water these women are expected to fill with their routines. 'Small wonder their arm movements appear exaggerated and larger than life when you see them on the small television screen,' Jackie Brayshaw of the Amateur

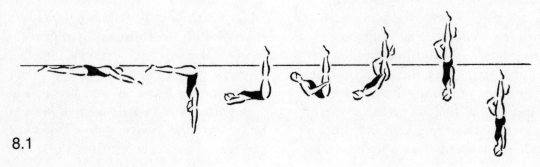

Swimming Association (ASA) Education Committee points out. Then, of course, there's the dreaded smile, source of many a scoff from the sport's antagonists. 'It's simply a disguise,' says ASA synchro coach Debbie Figuerido, 'allowing the swimmer to breathe with the mouth whilst making the performance look effortless. After all, in which other sport do you perform such vigorous and prolonged exercise while holding your breath?' And the nose clips? Funny that competitive divers can wear them without comment, but the moment a synchro swimmer puts one on, people snigger patronizingly as if their use reflects some female inability to cope with the demands of the sport. So why wear them, then?

## A nose for action

Our noses efficiently prevent unwanted fluids from getting into the back of our throats, as long as we remain upright. In any other position, the water washes over the sensitive membranes there, stinging like crazy because of the difference in concentration with our body's natural fluids. The only option is to maintain a steady stream of air bubbles from our nasal passages (see page 74) to keep the water out – an impossibility throughout a long and complicated underwater synchro routine. Hence the clip, which has the added advantage of protecting the facial sinuses against changes in pressure.

## Skills with athletic potential

There's no getting away from the fact that while you might not agree with the acceptance of some sports as Olympic disciplines, synchro is an extremely demanding form of exercise. Watch it with

> A gymnast performing underwater ... A 400-metre freestyle event in swimming with little opportunity to breathe ... The water polo player's ability to emerge above the surface of the water with power and strength, with an added touch of elegance ...
>
> ASA booklet

fresh eyes the next time it's on TV, and try a few of the basic treading-water and sculling techniques when you next visit the pool. If nothing else they're great fun, and while it's arguably stretching a point to introduce the sport into a chapter aimed at examining breathing and practising basic water-confidence skills, the ability to move through the water using hand power alone is in fact being used now in drills for all styles of swimming because of the 'feel' you gain for the water – the slight adjustment here, the tiny change in angle there, all aimed at using water to your best advantage.

So, following on from the breathing practices below is a short series of deceptively demanding exercises for a thorough water workout.

# Breathing and Bobbing

An obvious advantage of aquafit is the fact that breathing isn't a problem – although, as you well know, it is quite possible to swim up and down using back crawl and a modified breast-stroke without really getting your face wet. Indeed, does it really matter if you *don't* master the breathing pattern of a given stroke? After all, in terms of improving your CV fitness the important thing is that you are out there in the pool, gradually raising your HR into your training zone for about 20 minutes. Whether your face is submerged or clear of the surface makes no difference to this.

However, if you do manage to sort it out, not only will your technique improve so that you'll be able to maintain a strong, even stroke over a longer period of time – and without swallowing half the pool in the process – but your whole approach to swimming will change. The less your breathing interrupts your stroke, the more you'll get out of your workout, the more you'll then put into it and the more likely it'll be that you'll come back for more, and keep coming back over the months and years to come.

So if you still subscribe to the strictly no-face-wetting school of swimming, break yourself in gently with the simple practice of 'bobbing'.

## Bobbing – 1

In the safety of the shallow end in chest-deep water, keep both feet firmly on the pool floor, and hold on to the edge with both hands so that you know you are quite secure. Check your posture (see page 27), inhale fairly deeply, rise up on to the balls

> Even just under the surface at your local pool, you can feel the increase in pressure on your chest – your vital lung capacity instantly reduced by 10 per cent.
>
> From Thomas Reilly, 'Swimming', *Physiology of Sport*

of your feet, and now bend both knees so that you sink below the surface, making sure that you remain in an upright position rather than bending forwards or backwards at the waist.

As soon as you are under, begin to exhale through your nose. Gradually straighten your knees as your breath comes to an

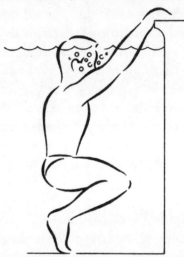

end, and, as your head breaks the surface again, inhale once more through your mouth in a quick but relaxed gulp before repeating the bobbing movement.

- Keep the movement slow and rhythmic.
- Stay relaxed and calm. You're quite safe where you are, and anxiety will only mean the muscles in your chest contract, making the action more difficult.
- Breathe in through the mouth. If by chance water does enter your mouth when you inhale, the entrance to your windpipe closes automatically.
- Breathe *out* through the nose. Water cannot enter your nasal passage if there is a steady stream of air bubbles passing out.
- Concentrate on exhaling. The inhaling will take care of itself.
- And don't inhale too deeply. That feeling you get where your lungs seem about to

explode is simply a result of breathing in more and more air without letting it out again properly. So try to keep your breathing as normal as possible. Over-breathing will tire you out very quickly.

## Trickle or explosive?

Believe it or not, you have just learned the basics of so-called 'trickle' breathing, principles which will prove invaluable when working on both front crawl and breast-stroke – not to mention any somer-saults or tumble-turns you may wish to try.

On the other hand, you could always try a bit of 'explosive' breathing instead, holding the air in your lungs while sub-merged and exhaling forcibly through both mouth and nose as soon as your lips clear the surface. Indeed, this is the type of breathing the top swimmers use because having a lungful of air during the propulsive phase of the stroke gives you a much firmer base in the water from which

to pull – not to mention allowing you to remain nearer the surface.

For now, though, continue with the trickle breathing above, and if you are already water-confident and wish to develop your breath control more, read on.

## Bobbing – 2

Swim out into deeper water so that you can't touch the bottom, making sure that a friend or guard is watching you, just in case. Legs pointing to the bottom, draw your hands down to waist-height with your palms facing the ceiling. Inhale through your mouth and pull straightened arms firmly upwards towards the surface of the water and onwards over your head as you press yourself downwards to the bottom of the pool (action and reaction, and all that).

When your feet touch the floor, push yourself straight up again, assisting your-self by pressing downwards with your arms

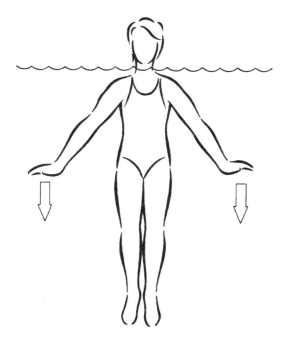
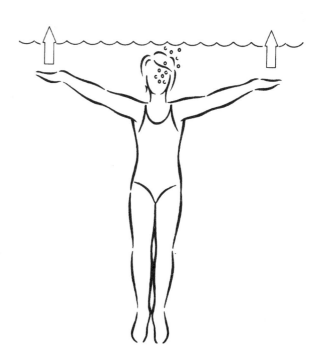

If your ears feel blocked on returning to the surface, the Eustachian tubes, which connect the eardrum to the nose, can be cleared through swallowing, yawning or forced expiration.

as well until your head breaks the surface, allowing you to inhale through your mouth once more. Practise trickle breathing as before – out through the nose as you go down; in through the mouth at the surface as you raise and lower your body through the water using your arms like wings.

● Keep your stomach muscles contracted throughout. If you arch your back when you descend, you won't work on the vertical, making your ascent to the surface more difficult.

## Bobbing – 3

And when you've practised this technique – and if your local pool is deep enough – try bobbing without touching the bottom, pressing firmly downwards using the arm action above in combination with a breast-stroke-type leg action to propel yourself upwards.

## Bob and swim

Alternatively, try bobbing down below the surface and, once you're at the bottom, draw both arms cleanly in towards your sides before sweeping them forwards in a breast-stroke-type action. Swim a couple of strokes under the surface and come up for breath.

● Maintain a steady stream of bubbles through your nose.

● Relax under the surface.

● When using breast-stroke arms, draw them round fully to each side so that they

nearly touch your thighs – an underwater adaptation to the stroke giving you greater leverage and propulsion.

# A Show of Hands

I noticed a swimmer take a very unusual breast-stroke pullout. At the end of his arm pull, he performed a slight sculling motion with his hands before kicking to the surface. He appeared to have covered a greater distance underwater than his competitors

Brent Rutemiller, *Swimming Technique*, Aug.–Oct. 1991

No, this isn't the latest in synchro developments but a method of increasing your speed through the water. Surely other styles of swimming are not looking to 'underwater basket-weaving' for inspiration, are they? Surely serious sports people have nothing to learn from all that aquatic acrobatics? Apparently they do, if coach Don Watkinds' programme of 70 unique drills and sculling games at the Bellflower Aquatic Club is anything to go by – teaching competitive swimmers about

Some of our sculling drills work the cardiovascular system. The tag games may last for 20 to 30 minutes. The swimmers are really tired afterwards.

Don Watkinds, *Swimming Technique*, Aug.–Oct. 1991

the subtleties of hand position and angles of attack, and helping them win races using a fraction of the hours normally spent training at this level.

## Sculling

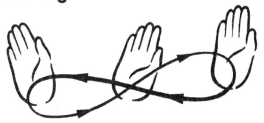

Sculling is basically an inward – outward motion of the fingers, 'labouring to and fro like the fin of a fish' (Digby, 1587) to create lift, propulsion and support. It's the closest we can come to rotating our hands propeller-style in the water, and is a useful skill to acquire whether you are a top-class athlete or simply having fun manoeuvring your way around the pool.

> If you find the action difficult, however, think about it a different way. Still imagining a figure-of-eight shape, let your thumbs trace the first loop, your little fingers the second as your palms tilt gently outwards and inwards as you propel yourself along.

## Standard scull – head first

From the back float position (see page 20), but with arms fairly close to your sides, bend your wrists back so that your palms face your toes, and trace a

> For these and every other exercise or stroke practice in the book, the important part is *feeling* where your hands or feet should be in the water rather than *knowing* where to place them.

figure-of-eight pattern through the water, leading with the wrists and sweeping them outwards and inwards to just wide of your shoulders and back again – about a foot or so and no more. You'll move gently forwards head first. (See drawing above.)

● Keep your head and neck in line, elbows at waist-level, hands near your hips and hips lifted.
● Keep your fingers closed for maximum push against the water.
● Get used to 'feeling' the water pressure to keep your propulsion constant.
● Keep your wrists and elbows relaxed, sweeping your hands out – in – out – in.
● Concentrate on the *outward* sweep, making sure the returning action works for you as well, rather than simply recovering to your sides.
● Never let your hands break the surface of the water.

## Reverse scull – feet first

Now, from the same basic position as above, bend your wrists the other way so that your palms face your head, fingers down, and repeat the sweeping figure-of-eight movement from the elbows, this time leading from your

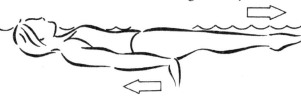

fingers to move yourself gently through the water feet first.

● As above, but concentrating on the *inwards* sweep more this time as your palms move towards you.

---

Get a feel for what you're doing as you push the water *away* from the direction in which you want to move.

---

## Torpedo scull – feet first

Now for one of the fastest sculling actions

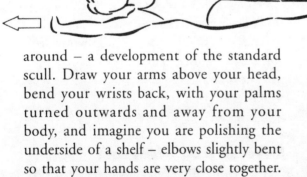

around – a development of the standard scull. Draw your arms above your head, bend your wrists back, with your palms turned outwards and away from your body, and imagine you are polishing the underside of a shelf – elbows slightly bent so that your hands are very close together. Trace your figure-of-eight pattern again as you move gently forwards feet-first … and be prepared to get a mouthful when you first try, because it's all too easy to sink below the surface!

● As with the standard feet-first scull above, but making sure your abdominal muscles are much more contracted and that you've got a good lungful of air inside

you so that your chest is well lifted.

Try this with a float between your ankles to begin with.

## The tub

When it's written out in detail, you might think that the tub takes a lot of concentration, with one hand sculling in one direction, the other in reverse to send you spinning gently round in circles like a record on a record player. (See drawing at bottom of page.)

But it's really not that complicated when you actually get into the water because you'll find you do it almost instinctively once you begin to feel the effect your hands are having.

So from the same basic position on your back – arms down by your sides – imagine you are sitting down so that you carefully draw both knees in towards your chest as your hips sink downwards, thighs vertical, with the tops of your feet, shins and knees resting at the surface of the water. Now bend your right wrist downwards so that the palm faces your head, and your left wrist back so that the palm faces your feet, and sweep both hands through their respective figure-of-eight movements as you turn anti-clockwise in this 'seated' position through the water. Now reverse

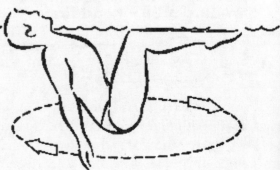

With all the above exercises, take care if you have any problems with your wrists or forearms. Don't over-do it either if you aren't used to the type of sweeping action involved, because it won't take long before your muscles begin to tire.

the action – left palm facing your head and right palm facing your feet – spinning slowly around clockwise.
● Keep your head in line with your neck and body by pressing it back against the water.
● Keep your feet high and hips low.
● Make sure your sculling action is smooth and continuous.

If you have difficulty actually getting into the tub position, though, try it at the edge of the pool with your feet supported by the gutter.

### Flat scull

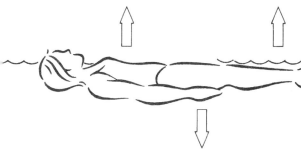

And finally, in many ways the most difficult sculling action – again from the same position, but this time with your hands flat and palms facing the bottom of the pool as you trace the figure-of-eight pattern. You *should* stay poised where you are, the amount of support you achieve being dependent on the speed with which you sweep those hands.
● Lift your little finger on the outward

loop, your thumb on the way back.
● If you feel your legs beginning to drop, sweep your hands further down towards your feet.

The deeper the hand position from which you scull, the greater the upward thrust and the more stability you'll achieve.

# Back on the Treadmill

Treading water is an essential skill to learn for water safety – precisely the reason it's one of the first things you learn at school or at classes in your local pool. However, treading water is not just about averting a crisis. Take away the arm action and it's an excellent tool for improving your level of fitness. After all, relying on the large muscle groups in the legs is very demanding once you hit the water, building up muscular endurance as well as really working your heart.

Make sure you keep an eye on your HR as you try out the next few exercises and kick your way to safety, strength and tone.

### Leg power

Throughout the following exercises, use the flat sculling action with your hands about 8 inches (20 cm) below the surface. Palms down and wrists flat, it will give you added lift and stability. And should you ever get into difficulty in open water, tilt your head back so that it rests against the water, bringing your nose and mouth higher.

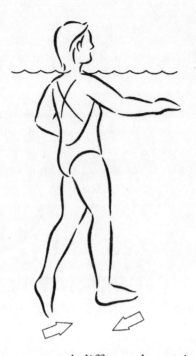

There are several different leg actions you can use to maintain a steady upright position in the water, the main ones being:

● a *crawl-type* kick: with straight legs and working from the hip, using your feet like paddles, toes pointing inwards slightly, for maximum pressure against the water.

● a *pedalling* action: as if riding a bike, and flexing and pointing your feet as your legs work round and round. Good for stroke practice. (See fig. 1.)

● a *side-stroke*, scissor-type kick: the lower part of the legs relaxed and really whipping against the water, toes again turned inwards slightly. (See fig. 2.)

● a *breast-stroke-type* action: squeezing the inner thighs and inside edge of both the calves and feet together. Again, good for stroke practice. (See fig. 3.)

● an *egg-beater* action: described below.

The last three are the most effective, but try out all of them for a minute or so each, and always keep the leg action constant and even so that your body is balanced, your breathing regular and relaxed. As your skill improves, the demand they place on your CV system will gradually start to decrease. So when you feel it getting easier, have a go at the progressions below and increase the length of time you spend on each as you burn up those calories.

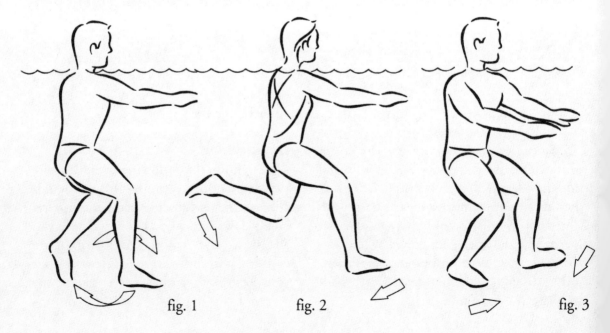

fig. 1          fig. 2          fig. 3

## The egg-beater

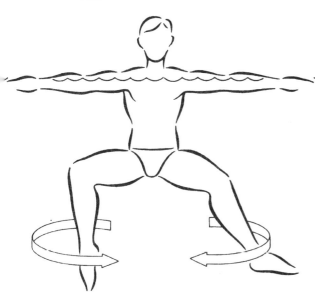

This method of treading water is basically a development from the simple breast-stroke method, except your legs are out of synch to give yourself continuous support and lift in the water.

To begin with, sit on the poolside, legs apart and knees bent, and circle your lower legs alternately inwards – left foot moving clockwise, right foot moving anti-clockwise – with your ankles and toes flexing and pointing as they move round and round.

Now slip into the pool and begin working with the breast-stroke leg action above, before gradually working the legs in opposition as you try to whip those feet around inwards.

● Keep your upper body relaxed and lifted. If anything, lean slightly back and keep your chin raised a fraction.
● Stay seated. Your thighs should remain at 90° to your body throughout the movement so that they are parallel to the surface.

● Keep your knees wide, but always comfortable.
● Work those ankles. Flex them as they circle forwards; point them as they follow through to the back.

## Progressions

And once you are happy treading water in all these ways, gradually ease back on the hand action – first placing your hands on your hips, then folding them across your chest just under the surface of the water, and finally resting your fingertips gently by the sides of your head. You'll probably find it easiest with the simple breast-stroke leg action, but when you can do it successfully with the crawl-type legs, you know that you have really got it licked.

## Water-wheel

And before winding up with the short routine below, try the water-wheel, revolving you round and round like the tub you practised above, but this time using pedal-power instead.

Beginning once more from the back float position, twist gently at the waist so

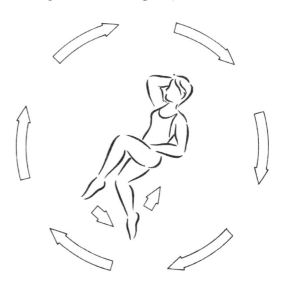

that you drop the right hip over to the side while keeping your shoulders flat and head and neck in line. Now, imagining that your head is at the centre of a record and your feet are tracing a circle around the outer edge, pedal your legs quickly so that you gradually spin round and round, sculling with your hands to begin with for a bit of extra support. Repeat on the other side.

● Keep your feet, legs and hips as close to the surface as you can.

● Point your toes when pushing your feet away from you; draw your toes in towards your shins when returning again.

● Keep the head and shoulders well pressed back so that your ears stay under the surface.

● Keep breathing steadily, and try to remain as relaxed as possible in the water.

## Progression

And once you've mastered the basic action

> Remember: you'll get more out of your aquatic workout the more at home you are in and under the water, and the better the 'feel' you have for what makes you move around in it.

… take away the hands so that you rely on pedal-power alone.

# The Hand and Leg Power Workout

Repeat each action for about 10–20 seconds each, building this up gradually over the coming weeks.

1. Standard scull, head-first.
2. The tub.
3. Reverse scull, feet-first.
4. Drop the feet and tread water, crawl-type kick - flat scull with hands.
5. Tread water, scissor-type kick – hands on waist.
6. Tread water, breast-stroke kick – arms folded just below the surface.
7. Torpedo scull or standard scull, head first.
8. Water-wheel right – sculling with hands.
9. Water-wheel left – no hands.
10. Drop the feet once more, and bob and swim for a few strokes before coming up to the surface.

# Chapter 10

# 'THE SILENT STROKE'

## Breast-stroke and the Art of Symmetry

'He has a frog in a bowl of water, tied with a pack-thread by the loins, which pack-thread Sir Nicholas holds in his teeth, lying upon his belly on a table; and as the frog strikes [swims], he strikes, and his swimming master stands by, telling him when he does well or ill.'

Lady Gimcrack on her husband's swimming lesson, Thomas Shadwell, *The Virtuoso*, 1676

It's comfortable, it's popular, and, as every single book ever written about swimming will tell you, one Captain Matthew Webb used it when he became the first person ever to swim the Channel way back in 1875. Evolved as a means of sweeping away debris from the swimmer's path to prevent the swallowing of anything unpleasant, breast-stroke is now the slowest of the competitive strokes and vies with butterfly in terms of high energy cost. It definitely has some advantages, though. The strong leg kick adds more to your forward propulsion than in any of the other strokes, making it good for life-saving and survival swimming, and it's also the most symmetrical and most stable style of swimming, allowing you to keep your head above water if you so wish, not to mention letting you see where you're going.

Of the 12 distinct styles of Japanese swimming which evolved as part of the Samurai code, one was a form of breast-stroke used for swimming long distances in open water – and in full warrior dress!

## Body Position

As with all strokes, the main aim is to make sure your body is as streamlined as possible.

Your abdominal muscles must work hard to maintain a good horizontal position in the water.

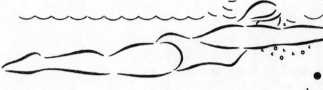

• Keep your head steady and shoulders square, even if you haven't got around to getting your face wet yet. Leaning into your pull on one side will make your kick twisted and uneven – and hence inefficient. But if your shoulders are steady and balanced, your hips and legs will tend to follow suit.

• Aim to keep your whole body in alignment. The moment you raise your head, your feet will sink and you will have to work even harder. However, to make sure your heels don't break the surface, you might have to keep your legs slightly lower than in other strokes.

# The Arms

Feel the muscles contracting in your shoulders and back as you draw your arms outwards, *down* and back.

Breast-stroke is unique among the strokes in that your arms stay underwater all the time. Most recreational swimmers tend to favour the 'straight-arm' style, tracing an upside-down heart-shape near the surface of the water to gain stability. However, this wide-reaching action does not maximize the full propulsive power of your upper body, so the following points aim to introduce you to the 'bent-arm' style used by the top swimmers – a style which actually feels rather short, almost abrupt

compared with the long, fluid motion of either front crawl, back crawl or butterfly.

• Imagine tracing an inverted heart-shape with your hands.

• Make sure you can always see

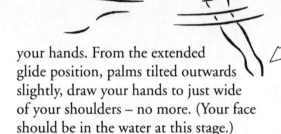

your hands. From the extended glide position, palms tilted outwards slightly, draw your hands to just wide of your shoulders – no more. (Your face should be in the water at this stage.)

• Dig deep! Bend your wrists so that your fingers drop, palms facing your feet, and pull downwards with your forearms, keeping your elbows lifted and steady as you 'catch' the water. The higher the elbows, the stronger the force, so keep your shoulders well lifted.

• Increase the speed and power of the backward pressure as your elbows bend. (Lift your chin.)

---

The biceps in your upper arms contract hard to draw your hands back.

---

There should be a 90° angle at the elbow joint at the end of the pull, fingers pointing straight to the bottom, palms facing your feet. (Breathe in.) You will lose power if you allow your hands to travel too far backwards, so keep the action compact.

● Lead with your fingers, palms turning upwards, as you curl your hands into your body and underneath your throat. (Dip your face.)

You can feel when you've got the action right because you'll discover some 'dead' water just below your chin. This allows you to rotate your wrists without encountering any resistance which might slow down your forward propulsion.

● Squeeze your elbows into your sides and extend your hands in a smooth movement. (Exhale fully.)

> The inward movement uses the pectoral muscles in your chest, while the triceps behind your arms press your hands forwards into the streamlined glide.

# The Legs

As with the stable 'straight-arm' pull, most recreational swimmers tend to favour a simplified leg action when it comes to the breast-stroke kick, tracing a flat diamond-shape with their feet to keep their stroke balanced and steady. However, as before, it only takes a small change here and a slight adjustment there to move your kick into another gear, whipping those feet together for added power.

> The quadriceps and hamstrings down the front and back of the thighs do most of the work in the breast-stroke kick, drawing the feet in towards the buttocks before pressing them out against the water again.

● Keep your heels slightly apart as you draw your knees in towards your body.

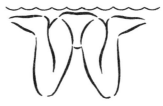

They should end up about hip-width apart. (Arms are pulling back.)

● Keep your feet bent out to the side like a frog, so that your heels are slightly lifted, your soles are uppermost and your knees pointing *down* to the bottom of the pool. (Elbows tuck into your sides.)

To gain maximum backward thrust against the water, your knees are much lower than in the flatter diamond-shape kick so that it almost looks as though you're making a W-shape with your legs when

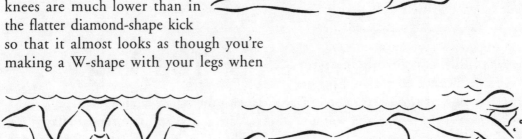

viewed from behind. Don't draw them too far forwards, though, as it'll make your body less streamlined.

● Keep your heels just below the surface. Too high, and they'll break the surface; too low, and your body position will suffer.

Breast-stroke is one of the few activities which works the muscles of the inner thigh, helping to strengthen and tone the whole area. Try five minutes of treading water using the leg action alone to discover just how little you normally use them (see page 80).

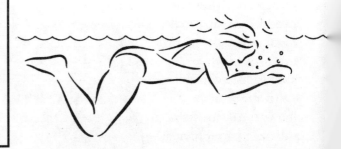

● Drive your legs backwards and apart in an arc-like shape. (At this point, your arms extend forwards.)
● Now concentrate on the inner legs – the inner edge of the feet and shins – as you squeeze them together again.
● Accelerate the movement as your feet

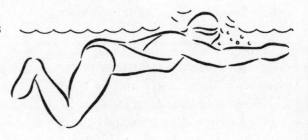

'whip' through the water. Keep your lower legs loose and relaxed for maximum power from the flicking motion.

● Point your toes at the last second to increase the paddle effect from your feet.

---

Breast-stroke makes good use of both shin and calf muscles as you flatten and point your feet for a little added pressure against the water.

---

● Pause slightly in the glide before beginning the action again. (Arms begin their outward pull.)

The aim of breaststroke is to achieve as near continual propulsion as possible by alternating arm and leg force: *arm pull – breathe – kick – arm pull – breathe – kick.*

# Breathing

If you really want to achieve good strong propulsion without making life hard for yourself, however, you have no choice but to get your face wet. Remember: if your head is up, your feet are down and the resistance you encounter increases enormously. So while the bobbing practices in the last chapter will have got you used to concentrating on breathing out through mouth and nose, the following exercise in the shallow end combines this with the breast-stroke head action.

Stand in the forward stance (see page 28) in chest-deep water with your hands holding on to the pool side for support. Take a deep breath and drop your chin forward on to your chest until you feel the water reach your hairline. Breathe out a steady stream of bubbles, and, when you're ready, simply

*push your chin forwards* chicken-style until your mouth clears the surface. Take another deep breath and try it again – face immersed, eyes forwards. Exhale and thrust that chin forwards again as you take another breath, practising it a few times until you feel happy with the tilting movement. It is a very small action so your head should hardly move at all.

Now try it while you swim.

● Keep your head as still as possible. Lifting it up excessively will affect your alignment in the water, and mean that your arms will fulfil more of a supporting role rather than powering you forwards through the water.

● Feel the slight lift your body gains when you press your forearms downwards, and use it to thrust your chin forwards chicken-style so that your mouth clears the surface.

● Take a quick and deep breath – but without snatching a panic gulp of air.

● Tuck your chin in again and look

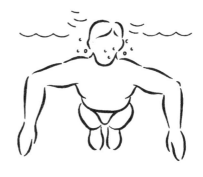

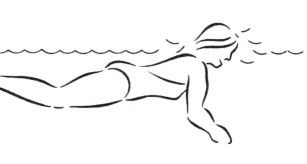

forwards to a point just below the surface while you start to exhale. Breathe out all the air in your lungs in a controlled way – imagining that you are blowing your hands forwards into that streamlined glide.

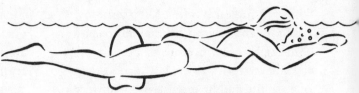

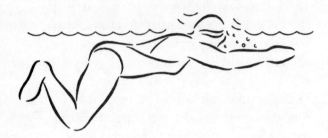

- Breathe once for every complete stroke. Top-class swimmers often inhale every other cycle, but at this stage you should keep the supply of oxygen to your working muscles as steady and even as possible.

Poor breathing is probably the main reason people get tired when swimming.

# Bit by Bit

Try a short swim. You'll find there's a lot to think about. So rather than trying to master everything at once, break the stroke up into its component parts after a length or two, and practise them all bit by bit.

## Arms only

1. Begin by practising the arm action while standing in the forward stance (see page 28) in chest-deep water.
- See how the angle of your hands affects the catch you get on the water.
- Feel the difference between firmly held

shoulders and high elbows, and arms which trail limply backwards.
- And practise finding that 'dead' water beneath your throat, squeezing your arms into your sides as your hands circle inwards and rotate before full extension.

2. If you've got a float, now try holding it between your thighs and focusing on your arm action while you swim for a width or two.

3. Alternatively, keep your lower half stable with doggy-paddle legs and again work on your upper body.

Go back to the full stroke for a while before focusing on the leg action a bit more.

## Legs only

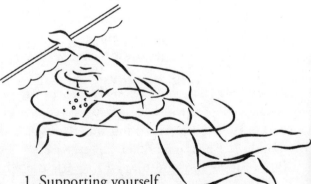

1. Supporting yourself with the bracket grip against the side of the pool (see page 28) – or, indeed, holding on to a friend's arm as he or she moves slowly forwards – trace the circling movement with your heels. Feet flat and toes out, press strongly back against the water with those inside legs, and whip

those toes together at the last minute.

● Make sure you don't arch your back, but keep your neck and spine in perfect alignment.

2. For a bit of extra breathing practice too, drop your chin into your chest, balance yourself with a glide where your arms are by your sides and exaggerate the frog-like kick by trying to touch your feet with your fingers.

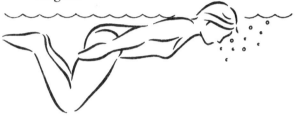

3. Roll over on to your back and practise the leg kick this way up. Keep your head well lifted and knees and feet low so that you don't have to think about breathing but can watch your leg action under the surface. Scull with your hands for extra support if needed.

● Really feel the water pressure against the inner sides of your legs and feet.

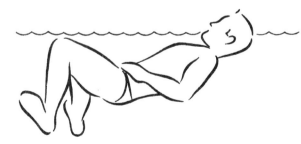

## Breathing practice

If you've got a float, hold it firmly in both hands in front of you and try steaming up and down the pool a few times using leg power alone.

Once you've found your rhythm, drop your chin, feel the water meet your forehead and synchronize your breathing with your kick as you push your chin forwards.

## Full stroke

Now put it all back together again – bit by bit.

1. Try doing two kicks to every pull, and two pulls to every kick so that you can still concentrate on all the different points.

2. Push yourself off from the side into a glide, head down, before pulling your arms back, breathing and kicking. Glide again, slowing the sequence and exaggerating the pause to make sure your alignment is good and to feel the power of your kick drive you forwards.

3. And finally, try a few widths of perfect breast-stroke, noting how many strokes it takes to do each one so that you can see your improvement as the weeks progress.

Turn to Chapter 13 for a swimfit programme.

# Chapter 11

# WINDMILLS NO MORE
## Back Crawl With Push

'[He was] so uneducated he could neither read nor swim.'

A Greek proverb quoted by Plato in his *Laws* – and a cutting insult!

It's readily adaptable into a variety of different forms. You can breathe whenever you feel like it. And taken slowly it's extremely relaxing because of the full-body stretch you achieve in the process. In fact, the only possible problem with the back crawl is that you can't see where you're going.

The familiar alternating arms and beating leg action were developed from the breast-stroke kick still used in life-saving today in around 1912. And like breast-stroke, back crawl has two basic arm movements: the straight-arm style which most recreational swimmers use, and the powerful bent-arm action used at competition level – not that difficult to master once you get a feel for the action. Here's how.

## Body Position

Once again, aim to lie as near horizontally as possible, but making sure that your legs are sufficiently low in the water so your knees don't break the surface.

● Keep your lungs fully inflated and chest lifted. This will keep you floating higher.

● Avoid 'sitting' in the water. Keep your stomach muscles contracted and hips lifted to the surface.

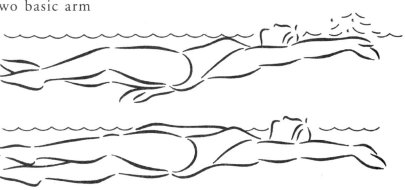

> The abdominal muscles control the whole movement by anchoring your position in the water. So work them hard and strengthen them up!

• Keep your head still and in a natural alignment with your body, allowing the water to take its full weight. Relax your neck completely, your ears just submerged and head well back in the water.
• Eyes up! Keep them lifted to keep your chin up, because if you hold your head too high by looking down towards your toes, your hips will sink and you won't maintain a streamlined position in the water.
• Allow your shoulders to roll as your arms rotate. Dipping them alternately will give you maximum leverage against the water.
• But keep your hips as square possible. To avoid your whole body rolling from side to side with your arm pull, use your legs to keep your body stable.

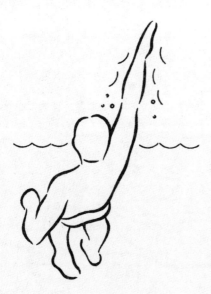

> Women-only sessions are now becoming much more frequent in local pools everywhere, a development which should be applauded. Not only do they lessen that feeling of self-consciousness when wandering around with very little on, they also allow women of every race and creed to benefit from this inspiring approach to health and fitness. And the more opportunity women have to exercise together, the better!

# The Arms

The arm action in back crawl is quite a complicated movement because it involves a so-called 'circumduction' of the shoulder joint – in other words, your arms almost trace a full circle. And while you may not be able to feel them working individually for a while, you are actually using the muscles capping the shoulders (deltoids), those in the upper-arm (biceps and triceps), the pectorals forming a type of armour across the chest, and the latissimus dorsi down your back. Not a bad upper-body workout when you think about it.
• Keep your arm straight when it's above the water. Try not to lose power by bending your elbow before it's immersed.
• Keep the momentum. Don't pause before your hand enters the water but swing it straight over and in.
• Keep your arm in line with – or slightly wide of – your shoulder joint as your fingers approach the water

If your arms come down well outside this point because you lack mobility in your upper body, make a conscious effort

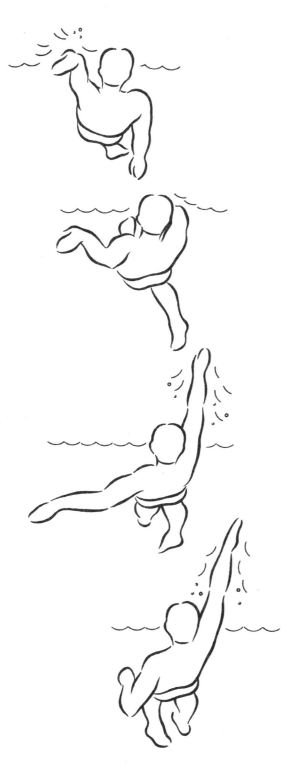

to squeeze them inwards, almost exaggerating the action to bring your hand over your head so that you brush your ear with your upper arm.

The mobility exercises on pages 31–2 will help develop flexibilty in your shoulders.

● Fingers, side of the hand and wrist slice into the water first. Your palms should face outwards and slightly down in a relaxed, straight-arm action.

● Small splash! As always, the action should be as clean as possible. Slapping your hand down on to the water wastes effort.

● Bend your wrist backwards, palm facing your feet as you pull your hand down close and parallel to your body, pressing it onwards to hip-level.

To get a feel for the type of action involved, stand in the shallow end with your back to the side of the pool and rest your hands on the edge, elbows bent and fingers pointing forwards. Now press downwards firmly so you lift your feet a couple of inches off the floor, before lowering yourself to the bottom again.

● Take care with this action if you have any problems with your wrists, shoulders or neck.

Now remember this feeling every time you pull your arms through the water, *bending your elbows* to 90° for maximum propulsion through the water.

● Keep your hand near the surface – a maximum of about 6 inches (15 cm) below.

● Accelerate powerfully through the pull and press.

About 85–90 per cent of the power in back crawl comes from the final push.

- Don't pause when your hand reaches your thigh, but swing it directly upwards and over your head again, slicing cleanly out of the water with palm turned inwards and thumb leading. Keep your arms moving continuously for continuous forward propulsion.

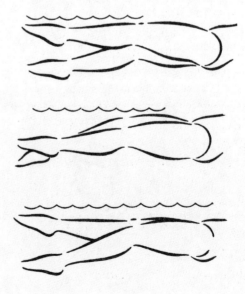

> While good mobility in your upper body will make your back crawl all the more efficient, the arm movement itself helps develop flexibility in your shoulders.

- Turn your palm outwards as it passes close to your ear – ready for the entry phase.

# The Legs

What can go wrong with a simple up–down kicking action used mainly for balance and stability? Well, while you might think that you're keeping your legs fairly straight during both front and back crawl, both kicks involve three separate joints – the hips, knees *and* ankles – making three areas of potential trouble.
- The movement can be too big or too small from the hip.
- The knees can bend too much.
- And you may not be pointing your toes enough to make your feet efficient paddles – flipping up and down against the water. So think about the action a bit before you start.
- Keep your legs fairly straight, close together and relaxed. You don't want to 'pedal' your legs so that your knees break the surface.
- Imagine that you are kicking from the hips, leading with the top of the thighs.
   The force travels from here to your knees, to your ankles, to your feet and onwards out against the water.
- Allow your knees to bend slightly as they reach the bottom of the downward action.

> Leg-kicking burns up calories. Use it just to keep your body stable and hips lifted in the stroke. Alternatively, lie on your back with a float across your hips and kick your way up and down the pool as an invigorating exercise.

> The back-crawl kick is excellent for strengthening and toning up your lower body, focusing mainly on the thighs and buttocks. The gluteals and hamstrings underneath you press alternate legs downwards in preparation for the powerful upkick in which your quadriceps and hip flexors drive your pointed toes back to the surface.

Your feet should reach a maximum depth of about 12–18 inches (30–45 cm) to pro vide the build-up for the more powerful upward kick.

● Become pigeon-toed – big toes almost touching! The water resistance will tend to turn your ankles inwards, increasing the surface area presented against the water – and hence the amount of force you can exert. Indeed, you might even find that your legs are one on top of each other rather than side by side.

● 'Shake your feet off' as you point your toes! It is the upward kick which can provide extra propulsive force, especially if you whip those ankles towards the surface.

● No splash! Only your toes should touch the surface – creating a mound in the water, not a frothing spray.

---

White water is wasted energy.

---

● And overall, keep the leg action even and rhythmic so that it sounds like a motor beating against the water. Simple!

# Breathing

With your face clear of the water, breathing is no problem either.

● Concentrate on breathing out. You don't want to inhale more and more until your lungs want to explode.

● To begin with, breathe whenever you feel it necessary – independently of your strokes.

● Gradually introduce a regular breathing pattern. Try breathing out with the pull on one side, and in with the pull on the other.

# Full Stroke

With arm and leg action fitted together, and even breathing under control, you should be able to slice effortlessly through the water.

● Opposite arm and leg. As your right arm begins to pull, your left leg kicks and vice versa – stabilizing your body for streamlined efficiency in the water.

● Count in sixes. Aim at six kicks to one arm cycle – three kicks on your right-arm pull and three on your left – although to begin with, two kicks per arm cycle will be enough to keep you balanced.

# Bit by Bit

And once you've practised the whole stroke for a short while, break it all down into its component parts again, concentrating on good technique.

> Part-practices are an excellent way of focusing on all the different points in the arm and leg movements. But when you put it all back together again in the full stroke you'll find that the arm and leg actions are slightly different.

## Arms only

The problem with trying to work on the arm action in back crawl is that it's hard to stabilize yourself and achieve a good practice position. You could, of course, hook your feet under the lip at the edge of the pool to keep you steady, but this is a lot more difficult than it looks, and at this stage I wouldn't recommend trying it.

1. Instead, stand in waist-deep water and simply rotate your arms, passing them close to your ears, turning the palms outwards, dipping the fingers and wrists, pulling down with elbows bent and recovering cleanly at the thigh as your palms press downwards through the surface of the water. It looks a bit silly, but at least you'll get a feel for the movement while improving the mobility available in your shoulder girdle.

2. Thumbs up! Now, if you have a float, lie on your back and hold it across your chest under your right arm. Practise the arm action on your left while kicking your legs gently.

However, to make sure you don't pull your hand down too deeply beneath the surface, stick your thumb up and make sure it just breaks the surface as you pull your arm along the side of your body. Practise this during your normal

stroke too, without using the float.

3. Now float on your back with both hands extended over your head, feet kicking to keep you balanced. Pull one arm through the water and recover it; then the other, pausing each time in full extension above your head so that you are really concentrating on the action.

4. If you have a float, this time place it between your thighs and work the arms in isolation.

5. And now try a width with one arm, a width with the other, and finally a width drawing both arms up, back, and through together – an upside-down butterfly stroke. Great to get those shoulders moving – and great fun!

Now try the full stroke again before focusing on the legs.

## Legs only

1. Practise the leg kick lying on your back – holding on to a float with both hands across your hips, or alternatively sculling gently with your hands down by your sides (see page 77). Try to shake your feet off without creating a huge spray, and keep the movement relaxed, leading from the hip.

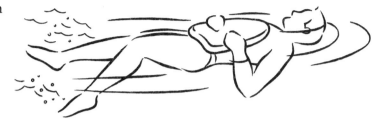

2. Now take away both hand movements and float, and see how successful your leg action is in maintaining a good body position in the water. Keep those hips high, lungs inflated, and don't let your knees break the surface!

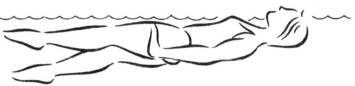

3. And finally, raise both hands above your head and repeat the movement – small splash, toes pointed, kicking from the hips and ears

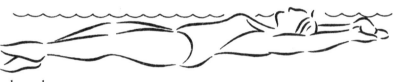

underwater. Round off your workout by putting the whole stroke together again.

Turn to chapter 13 for a swimfit programme.

# Chapter 12

# THE POWERFUL PULL

## Front Crawl Without Tears

'Their style of swimming is totally un-European. They lash the water violently with their arms like the sails of a windmill and beat downward with their feet, blowing with force and performing grotesque antics.'

*The Times*, April 1844, on a race between two American Indians,
and Harold Kenworthy who used traditional breast-stroke.

Front crawl. It takes only 70 per cent of the energy used in breast-stroke to achieve a comparable speed. Its simple alternating arms and beating legs is a natural action. And yet it causes more people more trouble than breast-stroke and back crawl put together.

But to whet your appetite and show you that there are some hidden benefits to mastering front crawl, we'll begin with a study carried out by J. P. Clarys in the mid-1980s. He looked at the muscular activity involved in the stroke and found that no fewer than *44 different muscles* have an important role to play in its execution. Of those, he focused on 25, and apart from finding striking differences in the extent to which each of these are used at recreational and competition standards of swimming, he also established an interesting fact about which muscles actually work the hardest when you use this stroke.

You might think, for instance, that because the main source of propulsion comes from the upper body, it would be the shoulders and arms which work the hardest. Wrong. Even for recreational swimmers, Clarys showed that it is actually the rectus abdominus – the abdominal muscle running straight down the centre of the stomach – which contracts the hardest, followed closely by the dreaded gluteus maximus in the backside. Without even thinking about it, you are working on two areas people are always desperate to shape up – and simply in order to keep your body as streamlined as possible as you move through the water. Fantastic!

> At competition level, front crawl is a good four seconds faster than butterfly over 100 metres. This, in turn, is faster than back crawl, with breast-stroke bringing up the rear.

So, with these thoughts firmly to the fore, it's time to crack front crawl as you swim into fitness and lean, toned condition.

much as your individual physique and style demands. It'll also help you raise your arms over your head again at the end of your pull.

# Body Position

There's no escaping it this time. You can't possibly attempt to master front crawl without getting your face wet. So keep your eyes open, look forwards and slightly down, and imagine how great it's going to feel when you actually get it right.

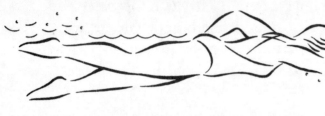

• Swim downhill! If you imagine this, it'll help you remain in as streamlined a position as possible, lifting your hips instead of arching your back as your body cruises along just below the surface.
• Make sure your head, neck and shoulders are in line with the rest of your spine. The water should meet your forehead.

> Lift your head up and, as with breast-stroke, your legs go down, the amount of resistance you encounter rises, and you end up using short, stilted strokes in order to support your body rather than power you along.

• Roll with it. To make sure you are in the best position for maximum leverage against the water, allow your shoulders to roll from side to side – not excessively, but just as

# The Arms

And while we're on the subject of arms, front crawl is not the frantic windmilling that people sometimes imagine. Far from keeping your arms straight, you actually dig in with elbows bent, your hands pulling the water backwards right underneath your body before momentum carries them onwards and outwards to be lifted cleanly above the surface.

• Reach forward deliberately, as if rolling your arm over a barrel. The most important thing to remember is to keep your elbow high and bent as your hand approaches the water, palm turned slightly inwards.

• Aim your fingers at a point approximately in line with your ear. Your hand should enter the water about halfway between your head and the full reach of your arm.

• Don't splash! Fingers, wrist and lifted elbow should slip downwards in succession through the surface, reaching forwards as far as you can once your hand is below the surface.

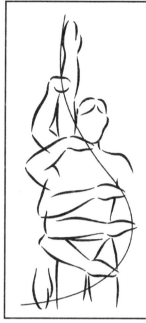

You use the muscles in your chest and back (latissimus dorsi and pectoralis major) to draw your hand through an S-shape pull from full extension, under your chest and out again at thigh-level.

● Catch the water as quickly as possible. Keep your elbow bent, wrist steady and fingers together as you press downwards and back, palm facing your toes.

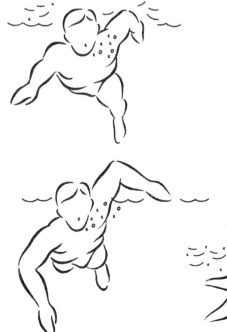

Your biceps work hard to bend your elbow and hold your arm in position against the water.

● Think of pulling yourself forwards *over* your arm. Hold that position so that your palm and under side of your arm face your feet as they pass under your head and upper body.
● Don't overreach as your pull comes to an end. Turn your palm inwards to face your thigh so that your little finger leaves the water first as your hand slices cleanly upwards.

The deltoid muscle capping your shoulder joins forces with the latissimus dorsi in your back as you lift your elbow out of the water and swing it forwards.

● Flash an armpit! – elbow high, wrist relaxed and fingers passing just over the surface of the water to swing your hand forwards to shoulder-level again. The main thing to remember is that this part of the action should be relaxed and controlled, disturbing the pull of your other arm as little as possible. So if you find the movement awkward because you haven't the strength in your upper body, let your hand swing out sideways more, tracing a wide, low arc-shape over the water leading with the back of your hand.

After all this, the leg kick is easy,

especially if you've already mastered the back-crawl leg action.

> Imagine what you'd be missing if you never had the chance to try out all these strokes because you were allergic to water, having a rare disease called aquagenic urticaria which brought you out in a rash at the slightest contact.

# The Legs

As with back crawl, the front-crawl kick uses three joints – the hips, knees *and* ankles, the latter helping to drive you forwards rather like in the breast-stroke by flexing and pointing at different times during the movement. The toes are pointed at the start of the downward kick, which uses the quadriceps and hip flexors to press the thigh down through the water. And after a moment's pause, the upkick begins. The knee bends as the hamstrings behind the thigh contract in conjunction with the gluteus maximus in your backside as your foot travels upwards, and you bend your ankle to work against the water before once more pointing your toes hard against the water pressure to repeat the action.

> It is interesting to know that, providing all things are equal, a disabled swimmer with no legs will swim faster than a swimmer with lame legs.
> Fionnuala Engesvik, *Swimming Technique*, May–June 1992

All that muscular activity just so that you can kick your legs up and down to stabilize your body and achieve a small amount of lift and propulsion! Indeed, if you're not careful your legs can be more hindrance than help because of the drag they can create.

Indeed, way back in the 1940s it was shown that to achieve a given speed using the leg kick on its own was between two and four times more costly from an energy point of view than using just the arms or the whole stroke. So control the action, and keep it small if you intend to swim any distance. Spend a few minutes working on your leg action during each session.

● Kick downwards and backwards from the hip. The action should be relaxed and steady, keeping your legs close together.

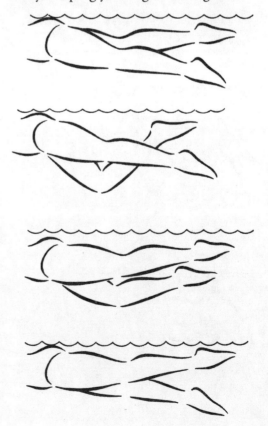

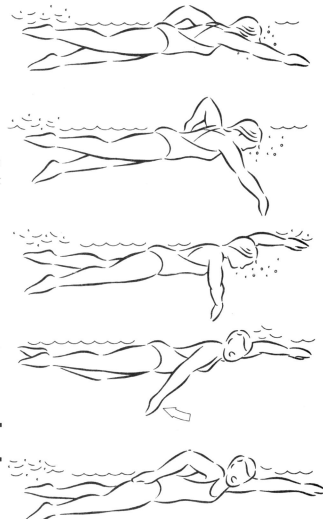

- Bend your knees slightly against the water pressure as they press downwards.
- Become pigeon-toed, feet pointed and big toes almost touching, so that you present the maximum surface area to the water and therefore exert the maximum force.
- Use your feet like flippers, keeping your ankles loose. *Whip* them downwards at the end of the kick so that your legs are almost straight at their lowest point. And while propulsion isn't the main function of the kick, a good flick of the feet will add considerably to the forward force.
- Press back upwards with the soles of your feet and backs of the legs. Bend your knees a little in preparation for the next back kick.
- Small splash! Your heels should only just break the surface. If you create a lot of froth, either your knees are too bent or your head too high in the water.

---

White water is wasted energy.

---

# Breathing

And now the fun really starts. How to integrate your breathing without compromising your action. How to avoid taking in a lungful of water. And how to last more than a few strokes before degenerating into a splutter of doggy paddle.

It's not easy. Some people find they prefer breathing on one side; some people are happy with either; and some achieve a balanced roll and perfect body alignment by inhaling once every one and a half strokes – 'bi-lateral' breathing, crucial if swimming in open water.

To begin with, breathe in as your hand leaves the water – although once you've experimented a little and established which side you're most comfortable with, you can always try inhaling a little earlier instead – during the last part of the pull. Start out with one breath per cycle (left- and right-arm pull) so that you don't deprive yourself unnecessarily of oxygen – again adapting the frequency after practising for a while.

- Look forwards and downwards to a point in front of you as you swim. Remain with your eyes forwards even when you breathe in.

● Turn your head – don't lift it. Imagine that you are face down on a mattress and simply roll your head to the side – ear down – as if about to speak to someone. Remember – if you raise your head, your body will tilt too much to the side.

---

Your head creates a small bow-wave as you swim, allowing you to breathe in without swallowing water.

---

● Inhale quickly and fully through mouth and nose. If you do manage to swallow half the pool, try inhaling a little earlier – before your arm lifts out of the water.

● Centre yourself immediately once more, with head and neck in line with the rest of your body.

● Concentrate on getting *all* the air out of your lungs when you breathe out – whether trickle or explosive breathing. The part-practices at the end of the chapter should help in coordinating breath and action.

# Full Stroke

As with back crawl, if everything fits together properly, you should be able to slice effortlessly along in a perfectly streamlined position – and without becoming a splash hit!

● Opposite arm and leg. As right arm begins to pull, left leg kicks.

● Master the two-beat kick. Although the top swimmers favour six kicks for every arm cycle, when you're learning to coordinate the full stroke the dangers of

---

Sometimes it's possible to learn good crawl technique more quickly if you ignore your legs. As you swim up and down using arm power alone, an effective kick may appear instinctively.

---

drag resulting from poor leg technique far outweigh the small propulsive benefits gained by this faster action.

# Bit by Bit

After practising the full stroke for a while, as always combine this with the various part practices below.

### Arms only

Beginning with the arms once more, these variations will help you fix your stroke.

1. First of all, stand in the forward stance (see page 28) in chest-deep water. Take a deep breath and immerse your face, practising the arm action in isolation for a couple of cycles before breathing again.

2. If you have a float, now try working on one side at a time, face immersed and float held firmly in front of you with your hand

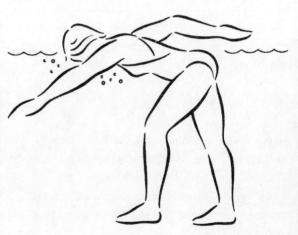

pressing it down on the surface of the water. Concentrate on extending the working arm in front of you and pulling it firmly back under your body in the S-shape movement. Kick gently for support.

An asymetrical approach like this is useful in focusing your attention of the passage of your hands through the water. However, it does feel different from working both arms together and can be very tiring.

3. Now try swimming with clenched fists. Not only will you notice the difference a strong, slightly cupped hand makes to the power of your pull, but it will also help to focus attention on your forearm.

4. Again with a float, try sticking it between your thighs and swimming with your arms only. If you feel yourself swimming faster, you'll understand the importance of streamlining your body properly – from the smooth entry of your fingers right down to a kick which provides stability and lift.

A pool buoy is a float designed to be wedged between your thighs to keep your hips and legs near the surface.

5. And now try both of these last practices but exaggerating the high elbow recovery by touching your armpit with your thumb as your hand passes by. Alternatively, swim close to one of the lane ropes so that you brush it with the underside of your arm when reaching forwards.

Return to the full stroke for a while and feel the difference your improved arm action makes. However, if the practices don't seem to have made things any better, continue working on your arms a bit more, and maybe leave the leg work until your next session.

## Legs only

1. Holding on to the side of the pool with the bracket hold (see page 28), float out on to your front and practise the leg action in isolation. Press down from the hips, whip the ankles, and make just the smallest splash as your feet rise to the surface again with toes turned inwards.

- Keep your eyes down so that your neck stays in line with the rest of your spine, and try to avoid arching your back.

2. Either with a float extended in front of you, or alternatively hands stretched out, one on top of the other – and your head up or down, depending on how you feel – work on your leg action as you propel yourself forwards. Keep your hips lifted, legs relaxed, and concentrate on the downward part of the action – an

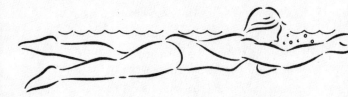

excellent way of burning up calories and strengthening and toning those hips and thighs.

3. Now turn on to your side, Superman-style – with one arm extended and head resting on your shoulder – and practise the legs once more.

And after you have tried a short

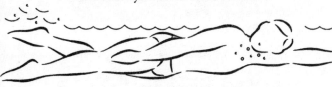

swim with the full stroke again, tackle your breathing with two simple exercises.

## Breathing

1. Back in the shallow end in the forward stance (see p. 28) as before, take a deep breath and drop your face into the water again, eyes looking ahead of you under the water, and hands supporting you on your thighs. Exhale and simply turn your head to whichever side you like to breathe in on – a good position to practise both trickle and explosive techniques.

2. And now swim widths. Hold your breath for your first crossing, then breathe once per width, then twice, then three times as you try to keep your stroke as smooth and uninterrupted as you can. A final cruise down the pool with all cylinders firing will test how your crawl technique has improved.

Turn to Chapter 13 for a swimfit programme.

# Reaping the Rewards

From the newcomer completing that first 10 m, to those among us with a keen competitive streak, we can all now reap the rewards of our success because The Amateur Swimming Association have an increasing number of programmes on offer to coax us on our way. For details of their challenging Swim Fit Awards and ever-popular Adult Swimmer Awards, contact:

ASA Awards Centre,
1 Kingfisher Enterprise Park,
50 Arthur Street, Redditch,
Worcestershire, B98 8LG, Great Britain

And if you're over 25 and fancy competing, dive into Master Swimming and race for pleasure right up into your eighties with other like-minded people of your own age. You never know, you might even end up swimming in an international Masters Championships in some far-flung country like Finland, Japan or Brazil ... Contact the ASA at their headquarters in Loughborough and add an edge to your training:

Amateur Swimming Association,
Harold Fern House, Derby Square,
Loughborough, Leicestershire,
LE11 0AL, Great Britain

# Chapter 13

# THE PLAN OF ACTION

## Swimming for Fitness and Technique

'In response to the fact that Ederle beat the record time of the five previous male Channel swimmers by approximately two hours, the press engaged in a debate over the validity of the old dictum that women are the "weaker sex".'

Cindy L. Himes, *The Female Athlete in American Society, 1860–1940*

It took Captain Matthew Webb 23 years to repeat his epic swim of 1875 and complete only the second Channel crossing ever. For a woman even to contemplate a feat like this at the time was remarkable. To manage it only three years later was an achievement indeed.

Gertrude Ederle was a supreme athlete. In 1924 she won three Olympic medals at the Games in Paris and had no less than eighteen world records to her name, confirming both her power over the short sprint, and endurance over the long haul. Her training programme can only be wondered at. But daunting though Ederle's achievements may seem, the principles behind them apply at whatever level you begin to swim, because while the intensity might have been considerably more and the distances involved much greater, her training sessions would have followed a similar format to the warm-up, pre-stretch, workout, cool-down and flexibility components outlined in Part One of this book. And just as Ederle gradually overloaded her body so that she could achieve that little bit more in the future, so the following pages outline two different swimming programmes, the first designed to improve the efficiency of your strokes, and the second showing you how to cruise your way to aerobic and muscular endurance. Each works at two levels, depending on your current experience and conditioning, and the Swim Fit Programme concludes with some useful pointers for those of you who wish to take your lap swimming a stage further. So read the material at the start of Chapters 5, 6 and 7 again before you begin, and relish the opportunities that taking the plunge can bring.

| COMPONENT | STROKE | | |
|---|---|---|---|
| | Breast-stroke | Back crawl | Front crawl |
| BODY POSITION | Head steady and shoulders square<br><br>Slight slope from head to toe | Hips high and chest lifted<br><br>Slight roll sideways | Streamlined and horizontal<br><br>Slight roll sideways |
| ARM ACTION | Simultaneous and symmetrical<br><br>Inverted heart-shaped pull<br><br>All action in front of shoulders<br><br>Pull out and down – elbows high<br><br>Smooth recovery under chin | Continuous alternate movement<br><br>Hand entry in line with shoulder – fingers inward<br><br>Straight – bent – straight sequence<br><br>Pull and push near surface<br><br>Clean, relaxed straight-arm recovery | Continuous alternate movement<br><br>Roll over barrel – elbow high<br><br>Entry in line with ear – palm turned out<br><br>S-shaped pull<br><br>Relaxed recovery – elbow bent |
| LEG ACTION | Simultaneous and symmetrical<br><br>Frog feet, heels slightly apart<br><br>Drive out – in with heels<br><br>Squeeze legs inwards<br><br>Whip feet together at last minute | Legs relaxed and close together<br><br>Kick from hip<br><br>Slight bend at knee<br><br>Pigeon-toes!<br><br>Shake feet off! | Legs relaxed and loose<br><br>Kick from hip<br><br>Slight bend at knee<br><br>Pigoen-toes!<br><br>Whip feet downwards |
| BREATHING | Inhale at end of arm pull – chin forward<br><br>Exhale during arm pull | Regular breathing | Turn head, don't lift – inhaling in trough<br><br>Exhale fully during armstroke |
| TIMING | Pull – breathe – kick | Breathe in on one arm, out on the other – opposite arm as leg | Breathe to preferred side – opposite arm as leg |

# The Stroke Improvement Programme

These eight-week programmes are aimed at improving your technique. The distances involved are fairly low, and the idea is to keep your pace easy and relaxed so that you focus on and perfect all the different components of the stroke.

Choose the level which reflects your current ability and build on that. Both are designed to be swum in 25 m lengths, although if it has been a while since your last trip to the pool, begin swimming widths during the first few weeks of Programme 1 before returning to the start and repeating the scheme using the full distance. Similarly, if your local pool is 50 m long, cut the number of lengths in half.

As the preceding chapters have shown, however, a lot goes into making the different parts of your body work together effectively in each stroke, so whether you decide to build on breast-stroke, front crawl or back crawl, your sessions will be a

| Programme 1 (25 m lengths) | | | | | | | | | | | |
|---|---|---|---|---|---|---|---|---|---|---|---|
| No. of weeks | Week 1 | | | Week 2 | | | Week 3 | | | Week 4 | | |
| No. of sessions | 1 | 2 | 3 | 4 | 5 | 6 | 7 | 8 | 9 | 10 | 11 | 12 |
| Swim | 2 | 2 | 2 | 3 | 3 | 3 | 3 | 3 | 3 | 4 | 4 | 4 |
| Pull | 2 | 2 | 2 | 2 | 2 | 2 | 3 | 3 | 3 | 3 | 3 | 3 |
| Swim | 2 | 2 | 2 | 2 | 2 | 2 | 3 | 3 | 3 | 3 | 3 | 3 |
| Kick | 2 | 2 | 2 | 2 | 2 | 2 | 3 | 3 | 3 | 3 | 3 | 3 |
| Swim | 2 | 2 | 2 | 3 | 3 | 3 | 3 | 3 | 3 | 4 | 4 | 4 |
| Distance (m) | 250 | 250 | 250 | 300 | 300 | 300 | 375 | 375 | 375 | 400 | 400 | 400 |
| No. of weeks | Week 5 | | | Week 6 | | | Week 7 | | | Week 8 | | |
| No. of sessions | 13 | 14 | 15 | 16 | 17 | 18 | 19 | 20 | 21 | 22 | 23 | 24 |
| Swim | 5 | 5 | 5 | 5 | 5 | 5 | 6 | 6 | 6 | 6 | 6 | 6 |
| Pull | 3 | 3 | 3 | 4 | 4 | 4 | 4 | 4 | 4 | 5 | 5 | 6 |
| Swim | 3 | 3 | 3 | 4 | 4 | 4 | 4 | 4 | 4 | 5 | 5 | 6 |
| Kick | 3 | 3 | 3 | 4 | 4 | 4 | 4 | 4 | 4 | 5 | 5 | 6 |
| Swim | 5 | 5 | 5 | 5 | 5 | 5 | 6 | 6 | 6 | 6 | 6 | 6 |
| Distance (m) | 475 | 475 | 475 | 550 | 550 | 550 | 600 | 600 | 600 | 675 | 675 | 750 |

*Keep a record of the number of strokes it takes to complete the last length each time so that you can see how much your technique is improving.*

| Programme 2 (25 m lengths) | | | | | | | | | | | |
|---|---|---|---|---|---|---|---|---|---|---|---|
| No. of weeks | Week 1 | | | Week 2 | | | Week 3 | | | Week 4 | | |
| No. of sessions | 1 | 2 | 3 | 4 | 5 | 6 | 7 | 8 | 9 | 10 | 11 | 12 |
| Swim | 4 | 4 | 4 | 5 | 5 | 6 | 6 | 6 | 6 | 7 | 7 | 7 |
| Pull | 4 | 4 | 4 | 4 | 4 | 4 | 4 | 4 | 5 | 5 | 5 | 5 |
| Swim | 4 | 4 | 4 | 4 | 4 | 4 | 4 | 4 | 5 | 5 | 5 | 5 |
| Kick | 4 | 4 | 4 | 4 | 4 | 4 | 4 | 4 | 5 | 5 | 5 | 5 |
| Swim | 4 | 4 | 4 | 5 | 5 | 6 | 6 | 6 | 6 | 7 | 7 | 7 |
| Distance (m) | 500 | 500 | 500 | 550 | 550 | 600 | 600 | 600 | 675 | 725 | 725 | 725 |
| No. of weeks | Week 5 | | | Week 6 | | | Week 7 | | | Week 8 | | |
| No. of sessions | 13 | 14 | 15 | 16 | 17 | 18 | 19 | 20 | 21 | 22 | 23 | 24 |
| Swim | 7 | 7 | 7 | 8 | 8 | 8 | 9 | 9 | 9 | 10 | 10 | 10 |
| Pull | 6 | 6 | 6 | 6 | 6 | 6 | 6 | 6 | 6 | 6 | 6 | 6 |
| Swim | 6 | 6 | 6 | 6 | 6 | 6 | 6 | 6 | 6 | 6 | 6 | 6 |
| Kick | 6 | 6 | 6 | 6 | 6 | 6 | 6 | 6 | 6 | 6 | 6 | 6 |
| Swim | 7 | 7 | 7 | 8 | 8 | 8 | 9 | 9 | 9 | 10 | 10 | 10 |
| Distance (m) | 800 | 800 | 800 | 850 | 850 | 850 | 900 | 900 | 900 | 950 | 950 | 950 |

mixture of swimming with both the full stroke ('swim') and part-practices ('pull' and 'kick') using a float and just arms or legs respectively. So based on the tips in Chapters 10, 11 and 12, focus on one element from the lists on page 108 each time and really concentrate on mastering it over the coming lengths.

## Warm-up

Gradually work your body into the workouts proper.
● Have a good hot shower before entering the pool.
● Easy swim: 5 minutes. Rest as often as necessary when you begin, but build this up over the coming weeks until you can

swim continuously for the whole time in a relaxed, easy pace.
● Stretches: 2–3 minutes. Choose from the selection on pages 52–7, although you don't have to spend as much time on this section as during your aquacircuits since your body is fully supported whilst swimming.
● Easy swim: 5 minutes.

## Technique workout

Select either Programme 1 or Programme 2 above. Work on one aspect from the lists on page 108 and follow the weekly plan. Remember: a problem in one area of your stroke may well be cured by improvements in others.

## Hands and Feet

Choose two elements from the lists below and work on them for a couple of minutes each to improve your feel for the water.

| Sculling | Treading Water |
|---|---|
| (see pages 77-79) | (see pages 80-82) |
| Standard scull – head first | Crawl-type legs |
| Reverse scull – feet first | Pedalling action |
| Torpedo scull | Side-stroke legs |
| The tub | Breast-stroke legs |
| Flat scull | Egg-beater |
| | Waterwheel |

## Cool-down

Gradually unwind before having a good hot shower and a cup of tea.

- Easy swim: 4 lengths using different strokes.
- Stretches: 2 – 3 minutes.
- Relaxing float on your back.

# The Swimfit Programme

These eight-week programmes provide the starting point for improving your level of fitness. As for the Stroke Improvement above, choose the programme which reflects your current ability, and build up your aerobic and muscular endurance through a gradual increase in distance and speed as your heart and lungs begin to work more efficiently, and your muscles develop strength and tone. Don't just stop after the two months are over, though, but develop this following the tips at the end. And don't look on Swimfit as an alternative to The Stroke Improvement Programme above.

The two go hand in hand, so if you are new to lap swimming, try to concentrate on your technique for the first three or four weeks and then begin to combine this with some distance swimming, adapting the programmes to suit your own goals and in a way that you can sustain over the months and years to come.

# PROGRAMME 1

## Warm-up

Gradually work your body into the workouts proper.

- Have a good hot shower before entering the pool.
- Easy swim: 5 minutes. Rest as often as necessary when you begin, but build this up over the coming weeks until you can swim continuously for the whole time in a relaxed, easy pace.
- Stretches: 2–3 minutes. Choose from the selection on pages 52–7, although you don't have to spend as much time on this section as during your aquacircuits since your body is fully supported whilst swimming.
- Hands and feet: choose two elements from the lists above and work on them for a couple of minutes each to improve your feel for the water while gradually raising your HR again and increasing the mobility in your joints.

## Swimfit workout

Aim to work continuously during this section of the programme as you gradually increase the length of time and speed of your swim. Your HR should remain steady throughout – at the lower end of your training zone (see page 17).

However, take short rests whenever your

need them to begin with, and reduce these as your fitness improves.

| Week 1 | | Week 8 |
|---|---|---|
| 10 minutes continuous swim | Add about a minute every session – or more! | 30 minutes continuous swim |

## Cool-down

Gradually unwind before having a good hot shower and a cup of tea.

- Easy swim: 5 minutes using different strokes, but concentrating on good technique by selecting one element from the lists on page 108 for each one.
- Stretches: 2–3 minutes.
- Relaxing float on your back.

Monitor your HR following the guidelines on page 17, making sure that you are never too breathless to hold a conversation.

# PROGRAMME 2

## Warm-up

Gradually work your body into the workouts proper.

- Have a good hot shower before entering the pool.
- Easy swim: 200 m.
- Stretches: 2–3 minutes.
- Fast swim: 50 m. Time yourself during this phase and watch your fitness improve.

## Swimfit workout

Aim to work continuously during this section of the programme as you gradually increase the length of time and speed of your swim. As always, monitor your heart rate following the guidelines on page 17,

making sure that you are not too breathless to hold a conversation.

| Week 1 | | Week 8 |
|---|---|---|
| 20 lengths continuous swim | Add 1 length every session – or more! | 50 lengths continuous swim |
| TOTAL 500 m | | 1,250 m |

Losing track of the number of lengths you've swum? Try counting backwards in twos

## Hands and feet

Choose two elements from the lists on page 111 above and work on them for a couple of minutes each to improve your feel for the water.

## Cool-down

Gradually unwind before having a good hot shower and a cup of tea.

- Easy swim: 5 minutes using different strokes, but focusing on good technique by selecting one element from the lists above for every length.
- Stretches: 2–3 minutes.
- Relaxing float on your back.

# Turning Up the Heat

What do you do, however, if you want that little bit extra from your workout? How can you still have a fulfilling session if your time is limited and you can't make up the distances? And where do you turn if you find lap swimming a bore?

Designed so that you can work at the top end of your training zone (see page 17) for longer than is normally possible during continuous swimming, interval training is a method of improving CV fitness and is used widely at club level. Based on timing and HR rather than increasing distance, the idea is to combine short, high-intensity swims where your HR nears the top end of your training zone (75–85 per cent), with longer periods of less intense work (60–70 per cent) which allow your body to recover. The ratio between such cycles of work and recovery can be as low as 1:2, even 1:1 if you're very fit, but for lap swimmers of good aerobic conditioning, a 1:3 cycle is probably more effective – 1 minute of high-intensity swimming balancing 3 minutes of less demanding exercise. Indeed, even the less conditioned lap swimmers among you can vary your programmes by using this ratio. Simply adapt the sequence a little to give yourself more time to recover, swapping every other intense bout of swimming with a nice and easy length or two: medium (3minutes) high (1 minute) medium (3 minutes) low (1 minute) medium (3 minutes) … and so on.

# Intervals Revisited

This 1:3 ratio is just one of many methods of interval training, using so-called 'active' recovery instead of stopping completely for short periods of rest to let your HR fall again. Why not try timing yourself over 50

> Well-conditioned athletes often use the high-intensity bouts to train anaerobically at near maximum HR. Stay within your training zone for now, though, and increase the number of cycles instead.

m for instance, and create your own, personalised intervals? The rest times should last about half as long as your initial laps, so if it takes you a minute to complete your first swim, begin each new 50 m repetition every 1½ minutes, completing a total of four before pausing at one end until your HR falls to the bottom end of your training zone once more.

# THE 'LUNCHTIME' SESSION

To discover how productive even a short session in the pool can be, why not try the 'lunchtime' workout for size – spending a total of just half an hour in the water.

### Warm-up
Easy swim and gentle pre-stretch following the guidelines in the training programmes above: total of 5 minutes.

### Interval training
Five cycles using the 1:3 ratio, beginning with 3 minutes of moderate swimming: total of 20 minutes.

### Cool-down
Gradually unwind and stretch out, again following the guidelines in the programmes above: total of 7 minutes.

# Part Four

# RECHARGING YOUR BATTERIES

# Chapter 14

# WATER THERAPY
## The Art of Relaxation

Most fitness books today acknowledge the need to take time out, giving your body a chance to take stock of all the new demands that you are making of it, and allowing your mind to unwind gently as you devote a little space to yourself. And what better way to do this than luxuriating in a long hot bath or bubbling jacuzzi?

Yes, *Taking the Plunge* winds down in the most gentle, most passive way possible by looking at the different forms of water treatment on offer, soothing your body and recharging your batteries while allowing you plenty of time to reflect on the amazing properties of this simple, inspiring element.

Hydrotherapy means different things to different people:
- 'the harmonization of the body and mind under the salutary effect of water'
*The European*
- the treatment of injury by physiotherapists using pools, jets and underwater massage
- any salon or beauty treatment involving water, including jacuzzis, and bathing and cleansing with exotic preparations.

## From Freezing Baths to Soothing Spas

What is it about water that obsessed the

'The chief virtues of medicinal springs are, in a great measure, owing to the Water itself, independent of their solid ingredients.'
Friderick Hoffman, 18th-century Fellow of the Royal Society

Ancient Greeks and Romans, and today absorbs hundreds of thousands of people in spas and salons the world over? Our thirst for hydrotherapy in all its forms seems unquenchable. Some property – be it a primitive attraction encoded deep in our genetic make-up, or a simple emotional response to a change of scene – *something* draws us irresistibly, almost hypnotically, to seek its restorative powers.

# Psychrolutes – or Lovers of Cold Water

> Every ailment, as long as it is still curable, can be cured by the stimulus of water
> Father Sebastian Kneipp, 18th-century specialist in water therapies

The Greek and Roman civilizations thought it harmonized body and mind. Muslims thought it helped find truth. And for Christians and Jews it cleansed the body and purified the soul. The use of cold water in various treatments has a long and impressive pedigree, boasting such famous exponents as Florence Nightingale and the father of evolution, Charles Darwin.

> The poet Shelley kept his head clear by drenching it in a bowl of cold water several times a day.

Indeed, the Kneipp Hydrotherapy Centre in Bad Wörishofen, Germany, has been offering a variety of chilly treatments as part of a more general health programme since 1889, and on a more informal basis a dedicated few continue to leap stoically into Hyde Park's freezing Serpentine despite the vagaries of the British weather. But it has taken recent studies into so-called 'thermo-regulatory hydrotherapy' (TRHT) by Professor Vijay Kakkar at the Thrombosis Research Institute in London to revive a more widespread interest in such cold-water bathing in this country.

> Cool tip for headaches: place a cold cloth or icepack on your neck while your hands and feet are immersed in warm water.

## Chill out

However, TRHT, 'is not simply having a cold shower or a dip in cold water,' according to Professor Kakkar in *The European* in May 1993, 'though these can be beneficial. It is a therapy based on a

> Cold water treatments like TRHT could help in the battle against certain heart conditions, as well as fighting colds and flu, brightening the complexion, strengthening nails, stimulating hair growth – even slowing signs of aging.

*conditioned* reflex, whereby the body is trained to adapt to a lower temperature at which an improved function can occur.'

TRHT is a treatment you can try at home, and consists of four distinct phases lasting a maximum of half an hour. You begin by walking around in a cold-water bath for three to five minutes in order to get your feet used to the temperature. You then sit down for a comparable length of time to acclimatize your lower half, before building up through a 10-day training programme to 10–20 minutes' total

> Shivering is a repeated involuntary contraction of the skeletal muscles designed to generate heat, the muscles producing three to five times as much heat when shivering as when at rest.

▲ Do not try TRHT without consulting your local doctor if you are on any kind of medication, or have a heart condition or high blood pressure. And if you do fancy following the full conditioning programme, the strict guidelines can be obtained by contacting Professor Kakkar directly at the London Thrombosis Institute.

immersion – neck and back of the head included.

Once the bathing is over, the idea is not to shock your system by any sudden and extreme changes in body temperature that are used in traditional Nordic spas, but to rewarm yourself gradually by dressing quickly (no warm-up hot showers here!) and taking in warm fluids and lots of carbohydrates. Over the next few hours you feel an amazing glowing sensation in your feet, chest, upper back and face as you slowly thaw out again – the glow probably resulting from a dramatic increase in your metabolic rate.

And exactly *how* cold is the water? You begin at a chilly 20°C and reduce this gradually to 16° C.

## The TRHT phenomenon

As with the more traditional forms of cold-water hydrotherapy like water treadmills, foot baths and wrapping the calves in ice-cold towels, TRHT improves the circulation and therefore the flow of oxygen around the body.

Initial research suggests that such conditioning could also be useful in the treatment of thrombosis and other circulatory and heart disorders by helping to counteract the blood's clotting mechanism. It may also boost the production of white blood cells – the body's immune system – and so have great potential for the treatment of colds and viruses, not to mention post-viral syndrome, or ME. It makes you wonder why anyone would ever bother to have a boring old hot bath again?

Cold baths *don't* shrivel your sex life! Instead, they may actually help to raise oestrogen and testosterone levels – with useful implications for male infertility and the female menopause.

# Turning Up the Heat

However, hot-water bathing still enjoys enormous popularity. At the other end of the temperature scale, turning up the heat can also be beneficial for the circulation. Initially rekindled by a Japanese TV series, hot springs – or *onsens* – have taken that country by storm. Despite their idyllic surroundings up in the mountains or on remote offshore islands, however, they are definitely not for the faint-hearted, since temperatures in the tub can reach a staggering 125° F (over 50° C).

It's not just humans who benefit from this latest craze: 'one *onsen* has enough bath space for 19 injured or exhausted horses at a time.'
*The Times*, 1987

## Bubbling baths and steamy saunas

Most people in the West turn to saunas and steambaths, though, if they wish to benefit from the advantages of steamy treatments. Jacuzzis, too, are a standard feature of sports and health clubs today – a type of whirlpool bath originally invented by Candido Jacuzzi to ease the symptoms of his grandson's rheumatoid arthritis. The idea is to massage the body gently while helping to relax the muscles, and this is why water treatments like jet showers, bubbling baths and hydromassage are widely used in the

---

Even horses have benefited from Jacuzzi's invention. Purpose-built 'horse wellies' are now available to massage injured legs – although some yards create a similar effect by using a bucket and vacuum-cleaner hose with the suction pump put in reverse!

---

treatment of injuries – and why they are so wonderfully enjoyable.

# Thalassotherapy and the School of Beauty

As long ago as the fifth century BC, the Greek dramatist Euripides claimed that the sea was a cure for all human ailments. Whatever the actual physiological or psychological benefit of this, sea treat-ments are currently undergoing something of a revival in Europe with the increasing popularity of thalassotherapy, or what one of its leading British proponents, Erna Low Consultants, describes as 'the use of sea water, sea muds, sea weeds and sands…[for] preventative or curative aims …'

Thalassotherapy was first developed on a commercial basis by the champion cyclist Louison Bobet in Brittany over 30 years ago and is based on the idea that sea water is comparable to human blood, containing a great many 'nutritive' compounds and trace elements, not to mention 'self-purifying' plankton. Floating or working out in sea water at near body temperatures, therefore, is supposed to 'facilitate the exchange and the penetration of the active elements through the skin'.

---

Skin 'nourishment' is scientifically impossible, since nothing penetrates the stratum corneum [deeper layers].'
Naomi Wolf, *The Beauty Myth*

---

It may be of interest to note some research by J. P. O'Hare and partners on the effects of immersion in Bath spa water (*British Medical Journal*, 1985). One crucial element in any spa's mystical appeal is the idea that water minerals can be absorbed by the body. But O'Hare's study found that this did not take place. A warning, maybe. Indulging yourself in expensive body wraps, and relaxing in therapeutic pools full of marvellous-

---

Reputedly in abundance around waterfalls and the sea, 'negative ions' are said to clear our heads, if studies carried out in Eastern Europe are to be believed. And while it is still unclear how the body detects such things (if, indeed, it can) they have been used in trying to explain some of the refreshing qualities of being near water.

sounding compounds will definitely make you feel better. But it may actually do you no more good than a basic no-frills soak in good old tap water heated to the right temperature. After all, you can always expand and moisturize the top layer of your skin with creams afterwards – creams which consist largely of water anyway.

# Thermoneutral Water

Question: Apart from getting wet, what is the similarity between flotation tanks, pools used by physiotherapists, and many spas?

Answer: Water temperature – all being regulated to about 35° C, at which point you feel neither hot nor cold but can hardly notice you're immersed.

Indeed, research shows that even sitting quietly in such 'thermoneutral' water can have a profound influence on our bodies. For instance, O'Hare's study also illustrated how such immersion not only helps reduce swelling – great news for anyone with rheumatoid arthritis – but can even help your body to work more efficiently by increasing your so-called 'cardiac output'. The amount of blood your heart pumps out every minute rises dramatically – not, as you might imagine, by beating faster as it does when you exercise, but by pumping out more blood with every beat. And on top of that the tiny blood capillaries also open up so that your periferal circulation improves as well.

Great effects, and all from simply adjusting the temperature of the water surrounding you. What happens, therefore, when you intensify such an effect? What happens when you remove the influence of all other stimuli – light, sound, touch and to a certain extent smell – by floating in a specially designed pool? In short, what happens to your body when you spend an hour in a flotation tank?

---

Eighty-five per cent of all illnesses are stress-related.

---

# The Big Float

> How retrograde, these masses paying enthusiastically to enter a state of 'sensory deprivation' in a culture where status is earned by frantically exposing one's senses to as many stimulations as possible (and as conspicuously as possible). The phenomenon fascinated me.
> Michael Hutchison, *The Book of Floating*

We pay – or get paid – to wind ourselves up. And we pay through the nose to unwind again. Extreme stimulation meets extreme deprivation, and suddenly the idea of lying quietly in a darkened room takes on a whole new meaning.

## The art of floating

The egg-shaped tank may look all very sci-fi and visions of *Altered States* may well spring to mind as you shower off before immersing yourself, but the whole experience is based on simplicity. You climb in, close the door, lie back, and because of the high concentration of Epsom salts in the water, you have absolutely no choice but to float. It is a completely dark environment, and apart

> Do not try floating if you have any condition in which the skin is broken. Cover any cuts with Vaseline before immersion, and avoid getting water on your eyes or lips – it will sting!

from the option of ethereal music playing quietly for the first 15 and last 10 minutes of your session to help you unwind and then rouse you again at the end, it's also sound-proofed. You spend an hour in a state of weightlessness, before emerging, limbs like lead and brain indulged and dreamy, to shower off carefully and head on back to the real world.

So what's the big deal? Do you get an out-of-body experience? Is your perception heightened? Is your life transformed?

To get the most from your float, go with a completely open mind. Don't consciously try to relax; don't stay there waiting for something to happen as this might have the opposite effect. Just lie back and enjoy the time to yourself. Indeed, it may well be entertaining to spend your time bouncing gently off the edges and spinning slowly round and round in sensuous isolation, but floating is not a cheap way of spending an hour, so treat yourself to seductive relaxation and save your acrobatics for the pool.

## REST and relaxation

Studies have shown that floating can initiate and help maintain weight loss, stimulate the immune system, speed up recovery after sports' injury and play a useful role in overcoming depression, alcoholism, smoking, recurrent panic attacks, lifelong shyness ….

Once you start reading about flotation, the list of positive benefits seems endless. Indeed, the body's complex set of responses to this so-called 'restrictive environment stimulation technique' – or REST – has already been thoroughly documented in Michael Hutchison's *Book of Floating* – and for those prepared to dismiss the whole area as very 'Californian', he approaches it critically, without any New Age-speak or psychobabble.

Along with the benefits to your circulation of thermoneutral water (O'Hare), lying down in a flotation tank lowers both your HR and your blood pressure as part of the effect REST has in reducing adrenalin-related stress. It also triggers the production of the body's natural opiates – endorphins – so that you quite literally feel good, and studies suggest that the increased blood-flow to the brain, coupled with a reduction in the level of activity required of it when the body is relaxed like this, allows your mind to operate more freely, opening up its more creative, more visual parts. Indeed, it's somewhat ironic to think about floating as sensory deprivation at all because your senses are actually heightened by the experience – your mind, temporarily at least, free to explore sensations normally overshadowed. It's also not too difficult to see how reduced stress levels could enhance learning capabilities as claimed.

But the question still remains. Would

> It's been estimated that nearly 90 per cent of your brain's activity is used to maintain your body's position against the force of gravity.

> Floating is a very sensuous experience, lying in limbo as the salt water gently massages your entire body and allows your muscles to relax more completely than under any other circumstance save floating around in space. It's much more effective than having a quick lie-down on your bed for an hour. Try it and see!

you voluntarily shut yourself in a tomb-like tank without light, without sound and in a state of prolonged suspension? 'Will I become claustrophobic? Will I be able to breathe properly? Will the door get stuck and leave me trapped? Will I drown...?' Remember: there is no lock on the door so you can gently push it open at any time. And you also control the light levels yourself if you don't think you'll like the dark, breaking yourself into the whole experience gradually if you wish. Or maybe you should try a touch of *dry* flotation.

### 'Dry' flotation

A contradiction in terms? You would think so. But the latest 'European Dry Flotation Treatment' is becoming increasingly popular – despite removing the sense of weightlessness so crucial to REST by supporting your body on a lilo or in a waterproof blanket. So in 1991 a study in the *Journal of Environmental Psychology* aimed to find out if such *dry* floats could produce a comparable level of relaxation to their older, wetter cousins.

Forgays et al. of the University of Vermont made two flotation tanks, exactly the same in every respect except for the all-important contact with water, and

although both forms of flotation did induce relaxation and a decrease in HR, the wet tanks were found to be much more effective in terms of both the level of relaxation induced, and the sensations of the experience. However, as the researchers point out, their dry tank was more sophisticated than those available commercially, and this difference may be compounded by the difficulty of trying to obtain a dry float which doesn't include all the extras – any complicated embalming rituals taking you further and further away from the thermoneutral environment, and further away still from the simplicity of water and skin. Nothing else comes close.

# Strictly No Additives

So it seems that 250 years before any detailed physiological and psychological studies into the effects of water immersion began, Mr Hoffman to a large extent got it right. The main benefit of medicinal springs and all these other forms of treatment does indeed appear to derive from the water itself. Germany's 150 spas are visited by a staggering 6 million people every year, and the health services in this and other countries like France, Austria, Switzerland and Russia recognize the validity of spa treatments and provide them as a state-subsidized medical facility. They even meet the requirements of insurance companies and the taxman! It's high time the rest of us went with the flow and immersed ourselves in healthy relaxation.

# DRIFTING THOUGHTS

'The most intense experiences were early morning bathes in Sydney Harbour, where the water was smooth, its texture silky, when swimming seemed like "an adventure into a different world"…'

Charles Sprawson, *Haunts of the Black Masseur*

What would you say if you found out that water was once a natural environment for us? What if you discovered that there's a closer link between man and sea than enjoying a splash or using thalassotherapy to improve your sense of wellbeing? The Amateur Swimming Association's *The Teaching of Swimming* rightly points out that 'Man is one of the few animals which does not swim automatically when thrown into water and has to acquire the art.' But what if this doesn't give the whole picture? After all, it's not as if we can speak at birth either, yet no one would ever say that talking goes against our natural instincts. And for a short time before we can even crawl, we do possess the so-called 'amphibian' reflex, a primitive instinct strong enough to propel us unaided a short distance in the water.

## An aquatic ancestry?

So, what if water's powerful effect on us and our imaginations runs deeper than the mere acquisition of motor skills? And would it ease any lingering anxieties we may have about taking the plunge if we discovered that we are actually far better suited to an aquatic environment than we had previously thought? Have you ever wondered, for instance, *why* our bodies are designed to be so buoyant and streamlined, and *why* our hands and feet can propel us so effectively through water?

---

About 7 per cent of the human race has webbing between their toes.

---

## A watery past

Developing the earlier work by Sir Alistair Hardy, the anthropologist Elaine Morgan took a fresh look at physical characteristics like these and asked why it should be that we are so at home in water when our nearest evolutionary cousins, the apes, are not. Perhaps the crucial 'missing link' in our development into humans had something to do with life amidst the waves? After all, the famous gap in our fossil records coincides with a time of

> Man did not lose his hair because he became an overheated hunter...[but] for the same reason as the whale and the dolphin and the manatee: because if any fairly large aquatic mammal needs to keep warm in water, it is better served by a layer of fat on the inside of its skin rather than a layer of hair on the outside of it.
>
> Elaine Morgan, *The Aquatic Ape*

enormous flooding in the world. Could we have taken a separate evolutionary path by leaving dry land for a while, perhaps, parting company from the other apes and monkeys and losing all our fur?

Indeed, the aquatic theory could explain many other features of our species – the fact that we stand on two feet, for instance, or that we can hold our breath and dive, sharing the so-called 'diving response' of other aquatic mammals (see page 71). And if that isn't enough, it could also account for the strange design of our noses, our poor sense of smell, how we developed speech, why we cry salt tears, why women's breasts are shaped the way they are and why we even consider copulating face to face.

---

Man is the only ape who does not fear and avoid water – the only exception being our shore-dwelling cousin, the able-swimming proboscis monkey.

---

According to recent studies, retaining adaptations to water could even account for many of our medical conditions, including dandruff, acne, asthma, brittle bone disease, varicose veins, hernias and shortsightedness! So whether we like it or not, we really could be natural waterbabies after all, adapted for making the most of this amazing, elemental medium. Why hold back, then? If you haven't yet taken the plunge, you're missing out on the experience of a lifetime.

# A Tale of Two Monks

> Aquaphobia, fear of water, is not inborn. Children learn to fear the water by watching their parents, their peers, or from their own water experience.
>
> Cinda L. Kochan and Janet McCabe,
> *The Baby Swim Book*

Although today it's sometimes hard to imagine, there are still many people in the world who have had neither the experience nor, perhaps, the conditioning to tell them how to react to water – whether they should fear it, or whether they should jump straight in.

A couple of years ago, medical workers in the land-locked country of Tibet visited the nearest stretch of coast down in the Bay of Bengal along with some monks from the local community. As the sea vista opened up in front of them, the monks went wild, stripping off and wading in, never having seen anything like it before. And while one contented himself with floating gently on his back after a little instruction from his watching companions, the other kept striding outwards, right up to his neck in the calm and tranquil water.

Suddenly, one of the medical workers

called out to him to sweep his hands about in breast-stroke style. And after much spluttering and a few tentative strokes, the monk began to swim.

# Come On In ...

Are you sure you don't feel like getting in? What do you need now to overcome your hesitations? Keeping fit by exercising in water is not new, and it's not a fad, as the quotations from Everard Digby over 400 years ago show. What has developed, though, is the range of aquatic activities you can now try, and this book hasn't even touched on team games like water polo

– the idea of seeing the SEA – of being near it – watching its changes by sunrise, sunset – moonlight ... fills and satisfies my mind – I shall be discontent at nothing ...

Letter from Charlotte Bronte to Ellen Mussey, August 1839: when she did finally see it, Charlotte almost fainted from excitement

and octopush (underwater hockey), or the skill of diving, the challenges (and exhilaration) of open-water swimming, or even subaqua – exploring the magical world of life below the waves.

It's up to you which approach you take. But come on in – the water's lovely.

# THE AQUACIRCUITS IN BRIEF

## Warm-up

*Spend 1 minute on each exercise.*

Pulsing on the spot
Water-walking
with shoulder shrugs
with shoulder rolls
Knee bends
Arm circles
Arm twists
Upper-arm action – 1
Knee lifts
Thigh presses
Space invaders
The grind
Side bends

## Pre-circuit Stretches

*Hold each stretch for about 10 seconds, on both right and left sides as appropriate.*

Upper back
Chest
Hip
Inner thigh
Outer thigh
Quadriceps
Hamstrings
Calf – 1
Calf – 2

## The Circuits

*Spend 1–2 minutes on each cardio; 30 seconds to a minute on each muscle.*

Cardio: water-walking
Muscle: heel and toe
Cardio: three-up jacks
Muscle: curl-kicks
Cardio: bouncing springs
Muscle: lunge – with forward push
Cardio: the skier
Muscle: side lifts
Cardio: jogging on the spot
Muscle: stomach cruncher
Cardio: back kicks
Muscle: side bends
Cardio: side raises – with downwards press
Muscle: upper-arm action – 2
Cardio: tuck jumps
Muscle: the squeeze box
Cardio: rocking-horse
Muscle: the U-swing
Cardio: water-walking

## Cooling Down and Stretching Out

*Spend 1 minute on each cool-down exercise and 10 seconds on each stretch – except for the hamstring and inner-thigh stretches, which should last about 20 seconds.*

Space invaders – arms bent
with shoulder stretch – 1
with shoulder stretch – 2
with triceps stretch
Knee bends
with upper-back stretch
with chest stretch
Pulsing on the spot
Waist stretch
Stomach stretch
Space invaders
Outer-thigh stretch
Inner-thigh stretch (20 seconds)
Water-walking
Hamstring stretch (20 seconds)
Quadriceps stretch
Hip stretch
Pulsing on the spot
Calf stretch – 1
Calf stretch – 2
Back float

# OPEN-WATER SAFETY

'Make sure that the banks be not overgrown with rank thick grass, where oft times do lie and lurke many stinging Serpants, and poisoned Toades … next that the water itself be clear, not troubled with any kind of slimy filth, which is very infectious to the skin, that the breadth, depth and length thereof be sufficiently known, that it be not muddy at the bottom …'

Christopher Middleton, *A Short Introduction for to Learn to Swim*, 1595

It was common sense in the sixteenth century, and it's common sense now. Nothing much has changed over the last four centuries when it comes to swimming in open water. We all know that there are far too many deaths by drowning in our seas, rivers and canals. We all know that just because a stretch of water is inland it doesn't make it any less dangerous. And we all know that if we want to swim outside the confines of our local pool, we must take extra special care. So here are a few basic guidelines to help you make that paddle in an inland pool or annual splash through the surf as safe as you possibly can.

• Make sure that children are always supervised near or in any water.

• Never swim alone.

• Only bathe in recognized areas where conditions are acceptable and tides not going out. A red and yellow flag means that the area is patrolled; a red flag means danger; and if a sign says don't swim – believe it!

• Make sure you know the location of any rescue equipment and the nearest phone box.

• Dress appropriately. On a hot summer's day the risk of getting skin cancer is even higher in water because there is both direct sunlight and the ultraviolet rays reflected off the surface to contend with. Waterproof sunscreens and sunblocks are an absolute must nowadays, and for outdoor aquatic exercise you might also like to think about wearing a broad-brimmed hat or bandana round your neck.

Cold is likely to be the biggest hazard in Northern Europe, though, sapping your strength and coordination, and quickly affecting speech and vision. So while a wet suit and insulated swimming cap are an absolute must if you intend spending any length of time immersed, always leave the water sooner rather than later, and wrap up well immediately you leave the water.

▲ If you get into difficulty in the water, stay still. The body loses heat between 25 and 30 times faster in water than in still air, and thrashing about or swimming around simply dissipates this all the quicker. Tread water quietly (see pages 79–80) with your head, neck and hands above the surface, and try to attract someone's attention. And if you do happen to fall in fully clothed, remember that your clothing will act in the same way as a wet suit, trapping a thin layer of water next to your skin which will warm up for added insulation.

● Never dive, never even jump into unknown waters – even off the end of a jetty. There could be *anything* lurking within – from rocks to rubbish, broken glass to rusty refrigerators.

● Always swim *parallel* to the beach, *never directly out to sea.* And try to stay in chest-deep water so that you can always put your feet down in case of emergency.

▲ If you do find yourself being dragged seaward by a current, never face it head-on. It will tire you out, no matter how strong a swimmer you are. Instead, move sideways or diagonally across it until you get out of its path, and only then head for home.

● And if you see someone in difficulty, THINK BEFORE YOU TOO SINK. Make sure that *you* are safe at all times, and if there is no lifeguard around, remember:

REACH, THROW, WADE, ROW, SWIM AND TOW.

*Reach:* if they are near the water's edge, lie flat on your stomach and try to *reach* the person, holding out a stick or pole for them to grab on to if need be.

*Throw:* if the person is too far out, *throw*

them something buoyant. If no rope is available to drag them back into shore, even a football may keep them afloat until help arrives.

*Wade:* if reaching and throwing have proved unsuccessful from the safety of the water's edge, think about *wading* in so that you are nearer the person when trying to reach them. Indeed, if there's more than one of you on the bank, you could even make a human chain: one person lying flat on their stomach again as an anchor, while the others hold hands and carefully edge their way out.

However, watch the conditions carefully, because if the water is too cold, too deep, or has a strong current, you could easily find yourself in trouble too.

*Row:* if this doesn't work and there happens to be a suitable boat nearby – one which won't sink, that is – you could then think about *rowing* out to the person. Take care, however, because they could well capsize you in their panic to get onboard, leaving two people in difficulty instead of one.

*Swim and tow:* even if you are a qualified lifeguard, only ever swim out to a person as a last resort. Whatever got them into trouble could all too easily affect you too.

In the right conditions, little can beat the excitement and satisfaction of swimming in open water. But it's all about knowing your limitations as a swimmer, and respecting the environment, so safety must be your one overriding concern.

# SUGGESTED READING

The list of books written about swimming and aquatic exercise seems almost endless, but here are a select few which deserve a second look, including some excellent handbooks for pregnant women.

Amateur Swimming Association (1985), *The Teaching of Swimming*, 12th edition. An authoritative little book which is updated regularly.

Janet and Arthur Balaskas (1979), *New Life*, Sidgwick and Jackson. Particularly good on the workings of the uterus, pelvic framework and pelvic muscles during pregnancy, with gentle exercises geared towards labour.

Janet Balaskas and Yehudie Gordon (1990), *Water Birth*, Thorsons. A gentle but appealing introduction to giving birth in water.

Glenda Baum (1991), *Aquarobics*, Arrow Books. A useful guide to aquafit by a physiotherapist – especially if you have a particular condition like back pain.

James E. Counsilman (1982), *The Science of Swimming*, 9th impression, Pelham Books. The bible, so chase it down even if you have to borrow it from the library.

Gillian Fletcher (1991), *Get into Shape after Childbirth*, Ebury Press. Endorsed by The National Childbirth Trust, this book provides simple routines and practical advice as your body returns to its non-pregnant state.

Michael Hutchison (1984), *The Book of Floating: Exploring the Private Sea*, Quill. A well-written and critical look at the research surrounding flotation tanks.

Carol Kennedy and Deb Legel (1992), *Anatomy of an Exercise Class: An Exercise Educator's Handbook*, Sagamore Publishing. A sound, common-sense look at all aspects of fitness. Excellent, so use it as a bench-mark for any classes you go to.

The Melpomene Institute (1990), *The Bodywise Woman*, Human Kinetics. Essential reading for all women, Chapter 4 provides a wealth of information about exercise and pregnancy in an accessible, approachable style. Highly recommended.

Elaine Morgan (1982), *The Aquatic Ape: A Theory of Human Evolution*, Souvenir. Thought-provoking and quietly confident, it's a book to change the whole way we look at ourselves. Watch out for anything written by this woman.

Charles Sprawson (1992), *Haunts of the Black Masseur: The Swimmer as Hero*, Vintage. Sheer inspiration, and a fascinating glide through the history and literary tradition of swimming.